Healing the Cancer Personality

By Barbara Carroll

1st Edition
© 2012

Barbara Carroll
Freedom To Feel Ministries

www.freedomtofeel.com
email: barbara@freedomtofeel.com

Edited and Published by:
Linda Lange
Life Application Ministries Publications (LAMP)
www.LAMPublishing.org
email: selfpublishing@LAMPublishing.org

Printer: createspace.com

INDEX

Dedication and Special Thanks 6

Foreward 7

Preface 12

Chapter One - Introduction and Overview 15
    Dr. Henry Wright 15
    Healing and Disease Prevention 18
    Several Parts to This Teaching 20
    Spiritual Roots to Disease 21
    The Studies - Cancer 22
    Are You Thinking Like God? 25

Chapter Two - Scientific Studies and Medical Proof ...26
    A Cancer Personality 26
    Personality Type 27
    Cancer and Personality 33
    Cancer from Unresolved Conflicts 35
    The Cancer Personality 38
    How Are You Reacting? 40
    Cancer Cells Definition 41
    A Life Changing Truth 45
    Think Sick, Be Sick 47
    God's Thinking 48
    Expressing Feelings 50
    Deny, Avoid, Suppress, Repress or Ignore 57
    Acknowledge and Deal with Feelings 60
    Personality Traits 62
    The Personality - Mind-Body Connection 64
    The Effect of Childhood Trauma on Brain
        Development 65

Will Childhood Trauma Lead to Lung Cancer?........66
Psychoneuroimmunolgy 68
God Speaks to Us About Our Health.................72
God's Study of Psychoneuroimmunolgy 76
Your Health and Thoughts 77
The Medical Community and God 87
Spiritual Roots to Cancer..........................97
Disease is a Curse 102
Character Traits..................................104

Chapter Three - The Great Exchange 108
Individual Personality Traits......................108
Living a Lie 109
Are You In Denial? 112
Inherited Patterns of Familiar Spirits.................118
Disease Prevention 123
Change Your Thinking..............................129
People Pleasers 132
Communication 134
Bitterness and Unforgiveness 156
World Research Links Cancer to Un-forgiveness...156
Bitterness 176
Passive-Aggressive Behavior 178
"Type C" Personality 180
Our Emotions.....................................196
Telling the Truth 199

Chapter Four - Satan's Favorite Weapons 200
Selfishness.......................................200
Entitlement......................................205
Covetousness and Lust............................206
Envy and Jealousy................................225
Evil Eye...235
God's Character of Love 239

Chapter Five - Cancer - After the Diagnosis....................242

    Cancer and Healing...252

    Healing from God 252

    Does God Have an Ego Problem? 257

    Manage Stress: Think and Behave Like Jesus 262

    Thinking and Vitamins 264

Chapter Six - God's Prognosis vs. Doctor's Prognosis 270

    A Healthy Environment 270

    Spirit, Soul and Body...271

    Broken Spirit/Broken Heart..................................274

    The Truth About Satan...275

    Disease Prevention 276

    DENIAL: The Ostrich Syndrome 277

    Chronic Disease 281

    Are You Past Feelings? 282

    Conclusion to Healing the Cancer Personality 284

Closing Prayer 288

Contact Information..290

References 291

Dedicated To:

My Father in Heaven who I am eternally grateful

Special Thanks To:

Judi Sweeney who encouraged me.

Dr. Henry Wright - The greatest Rabbi I ever had. He taught me about God and how to have a relationship with Him.

Anita Louise Hill - A dedicated and loving friend.

My two sons Geremy and Joshua - Who make me want to get up everyday.

Denise Walker for working with me on finalizing this book and encouraging me to complete it; without her, this book would not be a reality.

Linda Lange with Life Application Ministries Publishing (LAMP) who worked many hours formatting and editing this book for publishing and who has become a dear friend in the process.

Foreword

By Judi Sweeney

"I was shocked when I got a diagnosis of cancer!"

I had been a Christian (for over 30 years) and I was very active in understanding nutrition and eating healthily. I thought that I honored God and understood how to be a Christian. I thought that I knew how to take care of myself and my body. Yet I found that I had Chronic Fatigue Syndrome and so I had researched alternative medical modalities for healing. When I got a cancer diagnosis, I found that I did not like the traditional medical modalities that medical doctors recommended, so I was searching for other methods of healing.

During my search for information on healing, I read the book "A More Excellent Way[1]" by Dr. Henry Wright from Be In Health™, Global. I was intrigued by the book and I decided to explore the spiritual roots regarding cancer. I went to Thomaston, Georgia to attend a week long class called For My Life™. This class was an introduction to the concepts and the understanding of God and His word that would lead me to having an intimate and personal relationship with him. After attending the class, I was immediately healed from the Chronic Fatigue Syndrome. I learned about spiritual roots to disease from this class and I believed that I had spiritual roots to my disease.

Since God healed the Chronic Fatigue syndrome, I was faithfully trusting God to heal the cancer in my body, as well. After attending several more For My Life™ classes and conferences, and reading every book, listening to every CD in the Be In Health™ bookstore, I was disappointed that my disease was progressing. I then realized that a block to my healing was expecting God to heal me on my own terms. I did not want to do any traditional medical treatments, but in order to buy more time while I worked things out with God, I agreed to surgery.

The surgery went well, but a few weeks later I experienced excruciating back pain, and tests revealed that I had metastatic bone cancer that had eaten a vertebra in my spine. I also had evidence of disease in my lungs and liver. The doctor told me that I had one of the most aggressive forms of breast cancer and that unless I agreed to invasive medical treatments I had weeks to months to live. The doctor wanted me to have aggressive chemotherapy as well as radiation and other drug treatments. I carefully reviewed my options and I agreed to radiation so I could be able to sit and walk as well as have some relief from the unrelenting and severe pain. I received some relief from the radiation and I was able to get around some with a walker.

During this time, I was listening to a teleconference that was given by Barbara Carroll every Sunday evening. Barbara had also been involved with Be In Health™ for many years. She was teaching the principles that Pastor Henry Wright taught, but in more detail. She explained things in great depth and that helped me to begin to better understand the principles that I learned at Be In Health™ and that God talked about in the Bible.

This was when I really got serious with God and I wanted to know what gave the enemy a legal right to take my life. I devoted myself to praise and worship, studying God's word and listening to all of the teachings that Barbara had done for almost 4 years. I especially devoted a lot of my time to listening to the 14 CDs in the cancer series that Barbara had taught. These CDs were filled with the information that I needed to know. As I listened to the CDs I was convicted that there were many areas in my beliefs, my thinking and my behaviors that did not line up with God and His word. I listened to the CDs over and over again. As I listened, God revealed more and more areas in my life that I had to deal with.

My God was faithful and as I pressed through the madness of my life, He revealed to me what was not of Him.

With all my courage I went back to my past to understand and unhook myself from these unhealthy beliefs, thoughts and patterns of behaviors. As I listened to the CDs again and again, I became aware of the behaviors I had developed from poor coping skills that I had learned in childhood. As a child, I was trying to survive in a confusing and unsafe environment of alcoholism and co-dependency, and the abandonment of not being heard or seen and not being protected from abuse and violence.

I came to understand the depth of DENIAL, repression and suppression of all my feelings, hurt, and anger that I had held onto all of my life. This had created great internal stress on my whole body which affected my immune system. I recognized

I had lived my life performing for my self-worth. I had been a people pleaser so that I would not be rejected. I had many other co-dependent behaviors that kept me from having an honest and intimate relationship with myself, others and God. My life was a complete lie and the enemy of my soul kept me in the darkness so he could bring destruction in my life.

As I came out of agreement with these behaviors and renounced them and exchanged them with Godly behaviors, I purposed in my heart to learn new pathways of thoughts and patterns of behaving. I learned that I had to line up my thoughts and behaviors with God and His word. I also learned to be very aware and cognitive of my thoughts and actions. I came to understand that I was able to apply the truth of God's love, forgiveness and acceptance only as deeply as I experienced the reality of my pain of my past. The freedom I experienced was totally liberating and worth all the work.

Gradually strength returned to my body and much to my doctor's amazement, I was able to put away the walker. I have taken back my life and surpassed the doctor's pronouncements. The pain in my body went away which left the doctors more amazed.

Praise God! I can sit, stand, walk and even dance, I have no pain and good energy. The greatest part of my healing is the restoration of my relationships with myself, others and my God. The freedom that has come from walking out of these destructive behaviors that I was totally unaware of has brought me great joy.

The contents contained in this book and in the CDs from Barbara's ministry—Freedom to Feel—opened my eyes to the lies and belief systems I had learned as a child that did not line up with God and His word. Reading the other book that Barbara wrote called "Freedom to Feel[2]" several times until "I got it!" as well as listening to all the CDs many times, helped me to understand that kingdom which had held me captive all my life—Satan's kingdom.

My new favorite scripture is Psalm 30: 2-3 *[2]O Lord my God, I cried unto thee, and thou hast healed me. [3]O Lord, thou hast brought up my soul from the grave: thou hast kept me **alive**, that I should not go down to the pit.*

In summary, listening to all of the teachings that Barbara did on CDs and reading the books has helped me to really understand God and His word. They helped me to see the roots to the disease of cancer and to work with God so that I am alive well past any doctor's predictions.

Psalm 118:17 *I shall not die, but live, and declare the works of the LORD.*

Judi Sweeney
Virginia Beach, Virginia

Preface

Most of us have known someone who has had cancer or who has died from cancer. Just hearing the term cancer itself can evoke fear. Cancer is a disease that many people fear will "fall" on them.

During years of studying and learning about how our thoughts, beliefs and behaviors can affect our physical health, I learned that doctors and researchers know that there are personality traits that are commonly seen in people who have cancer. I found that there are many studies and articles written about these studies that contain a lot of information about these personality traits in people with cancer. After ministering and talking to people with the disease, I found that these personality traits fit in the personality styles of these people.

In this book I will discuss this disease we call cancer and these personality traits that people seem to have when they have been diagnosed with the disease process called "cancer."

This book is not only about healing from the cancer personality, but also preventing disease from ever coming into your life. When we learn about personality traits or characteristics of a person who gets cancer, we can see what characteristics to avoid and change in our own lives.

When people go to the doctor they are always hoping that he/she will pronounce them healthy. If we are sick and we have symptoms of illness in our bodies, cancer is the last diagnosis that we want the doctor to give to us.

Just hearing the word cancer brings on fear.
It is a disease that has some treatments, but
the treatments, very often, seem worse than the
disease. The treatments the medical community
has to offer are drugs, surgery and radiation.
There are many side effects from these medical
treatments. The side effects can seem as bad as, or
worse than the disease itself.

When someone has been diagnosed with cancer,
they can think that their only hope for recovery lies
with their doctors and their medical treatments.
However, most doctors will give the patient very
little hope of healing or complete recovery from this
serious disease.

Perhaps there is little hope of recovery with what
the medical community has to offer, however, there
is hope of healing if you add God into the equation.
There is definitely hope of healing when you know
the God of the Bible.

The Bible tells us this:

Matthew 19:26 *But Jesus beheld them, and said
unto them, With men this is impossible; but with God
all things are possible.*

Complete healing may not seem possible when
you speak with a doctor. A doctor who, is really
only a man or a woman, but with God, healing is
absolutely possible.

Romans 3:4 *God forbid: yea, let God be true, but
every man a liar.*

I know that God can heal any disease or illness we may have been diagnosed with. You might ask me how I know this. Well, I know this because I have seen Him do it. I have seen God heal people from diseases that the medical community has deemed "incurable." This book is all about how that "God possibility" can work in your own life.

The book was compiled from a series of teachings I conducted over several months on my weekly teleconference calls. May God Bless you as you seek first His kingdom and His righteousness.

Barbara Carroll

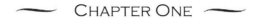

CHAPTER ONE

INTRODUCTION AND OVERVIEW

Dr. Henry Wright

In the small town called Thomaston in Georgia, there is a ministry called Be In Health, Global. The head Pastor is Dr. Henry Wright who wrote a book called, "A MORE EXCELLENT WAY[1]." This book has saved many people from living a life filled with symptoms of disease or dying with a disease that their doctors have called "incurable."

In order to understand this study about cancer, I recommend that you read A MORE EXCELLENT WAY.

Dr. Wright studied the Bible and mixed what he knew about God and the medical field and began to understand that our minds and our bodies and our spirits create one whole person. He teaches that you cannot just treat the body that is exhibiting a disease; you must treat the whole person.

Dr. Wright understands that there can be spiritual issues in our lives that can lead us into disease. He calls this "spiritual roots" to disease.

The Bible tells us that each person has three parts to their creation—the mind, the spirit and the body.

There are two scriptures that we can review that clearly establish that man is a triune being or created by God to have three parts to His creation.

1 Thessalonians 5:23 *And the very God of peace sanctify you wholly; and I pray God your whole spirit and soul and body be preserved blameless unto the coming of our Lord Jesus Christ.*

Hebrews 4:12 *For the word of God is quick, and powerful, and sharper than any twoedged sword, piercing even to the dividing asunder of soul and spirit, and of the joints and marrow (the body), and is a discerner of the thoughts and intents of the heart.*

All three parts of your creation influence the health and well being of the other parts.

The thoughts, beliefs and behaviors that you have will influence the health of your physical body.

Your body is speaking what is in your soul or in your mind and spirit.

The medical community has many doctors who actually know that this connection exists between disease and how we think, believe and behave. Here are some quotes from Dr. Don Colbert[3,4] who is a Christian doctor and author:

"I have found over the years that with every disease there's usually an emotion linked to that disease. And the emotion that so many Americans have is frustration. We have an epidemic of frustrated Americans here[3]."

"The majority of the patients that I see on a daily basis are over-stressed, and this contributes greatly to the illness or disease from which they are suffering. Our mind and body seek a state of peace and relaxation, which is called homeostasis. When a person becomes "stressed out," reactions begin to occur in the body that lead to the general adaptation syndrome. Unfortunately, when most patients finally come to my practice, they are already in [the] final stage of the general adaptation syndrome. I have learned when a person reaches adrenal exhaustion, we shouldn't just treat their body. We must also treat the person mentally, emotionally, and most of all, spiritually[4].

The connection between our minds and our bodies and our spirits is very powerful and real. Every thought or emotion that we have, can and does release chemicals into our bodies. Negative thoughts like fear, bitterness, hatred, revenge, or rejection etc., can release chemicals into our body which create an environment in our body that is conducive to disease. On the other hand, thoughts and emotions like faith, love and peace can release chemicals into our bodies that are conducive to good health and peace.

When we are dealing with emotionally and spiritually rooted diseases or symptoms, our disease starts in our spirit and our soul, and then eventually, we can see this as a physical disease that manifests in our body.

In other words, your body is speaking about what is actually in your spirit and in your soul.

Your body will speak and reflect what is in your mind and spirit.

Healing and Disease Prevention

The questions you may ask are: If I am sick, how do I get well? And, how can we prevent a disease from ever happening to us in the first place?

Getting well from a disease or illness that has already manifested in your body can occur as we get to know God and have an intimate relationship with Him. As we learn about the thoughts and behaviors and beliefs that we have that don't line up with God and His word, we can be replacing them with thoughts, beliefs and behaviors that lead to health.

Getting healed from cancer or any disease is a process. Dr. Henry Wright has called the process "Walk-out." We are going to walk out of our old thoughts, beliefs and behaviors and walk into new thoughts and behaviors that line up with God and His word.

We are going to be changed and transformed into new men and women in Christ.

2 Corinthians 5:17 *Therefore if any man be in Christ, he is a new creature: old things are passed away; behold, all things are become new.*

Disease prevention means that we would never get sick. It means that if we learn how to think and behave in a healthy and Godly way, we can prevent a disease from ever starting in the first place.

I want to make an important point here: I am not talking about positive thinking. There is a big difference between positive thinking and Godly thinking. Anyone can choose what they think is a positive thought. However, I want my thoughts to line up with God and His word, the Bible. I want to think and behave in the way that my creator says leads to a healthy life.

The Bible tells us this:

Deuteronomy 28:1-2 *And it shall come to pass, if thou shalt hearken diligently unto the voice of the LORD thy God, to observe and to do all His commandments which I command thee this day, that the LORD thy God will set thee on high above all nations of the earth: And all these blessings shall come on thee, and overtake thee, if thou shalt hearken unto the voice of the LORD thy God.*

God is telling us that in order to be blessed, we have to listen to His word and follow His word. Health and healing is a blessing. In order to be healthy, we have to be hearers and doers of His word.

James 1:22 *But be ye doers of the word, and not hearers only.*

I decided a long time ago that I want to learn all that I can about what makes someone susceptible to cancer or any disease. We don't want to wait until we have a disease in our bodies to deal with it our lives. Our best decision is to learn how to have disease prevention be a part of our everyday lives. The best option that we can have are not cures and healing. The best option we can choose and experience is that we don't ever get sick.

Every thought that we have can lead to creating the chemical environment of our bodies. Every thought that we think can secrete a chemical into our body.

What this means is that what you think and believe and do, can and does determine the health of your body.

The information that you will read in this book is to help acquaint you with God and His word and the personality and spiritual issues that might be causing an environment in your body that is conducive to cancer and disease instead of health.

Several Parts To This Teaching

The topic of this book is the disease—Cancer— and the spiritual roots and personality traits and characteristics that we can see in people who have this particular disease process in their bodies.

There will be several parts to this book, the first will be the information that I will present that comes from the medical and scientific studies that I have found. Next, I will present the personality and characteristics that a person may have when they have been diagnosed with cancer. Next, I want to relate those personality traits to God and His word. Finally, I will discuss the issues that come up after someone has been given the diagnosis of cancer.

We will also discuss what we can do to be healed from the disease of cancer. I will also show how the very answer to how to overcome disease, comes to us in God's word—the Bible.

Spiritual Roots to Disease

After studying the concept of spiritual roots for years, I am convinced that personality styles, characteristics of thinking and behaving can and do have an effect on our health.

I have seen this work in my own life and in the lives of many other people.

In this study about cancer, I am going to discuss those patterns of thinking and behaving that seem to be involved in creating the environment in the body that allows cancer to manifest in a person's body.

Sometimes we can think that diseases or illnesses are physical problems. We can think that if symptoms of diseases are physical then we should be able to get rid of our disease with a physical solution. I have seen people who have disease processes in their bodies go to medical doctors, shamans, chiropractors, surgeons, oncologists, psychic surgeons, psychic healers, acupuncturists and naturopathic doctors. I have seen people be managed by these modalities, or in many cases, I have seen their situation made worse.

I do want to make a point here—doctors can be invaluable. We need doctors to help us when we have an accident or an acute illness. Doctors can also help us to manage our illness or disease while we are working out our emotional/spiritual roots or the very issues that made us susceptible to disease.

Thank God for doctors when we need them. However, the true healing that I have observed have come from a relationship with God, our Father in heaven.

The Studies

I am going to begin our study with what the medical community can tell us about people who have cancer.

Cancer

As I have said, I studied this topic—Cancer—a lot. As I studied the disease of cancer and what the medical community had to say about it, I learned that the medical community knew quite a lot about the personality and behaviors that people with cancer seemed to have. I looked up studies that were done by people in the medical community that studied the connection between how we think and act, believe and behave and our propensity to get cancer.

I wanted to know just what the medical community has had to say about what the personality profile looks like when someone gets cancer.

I was very surprised to find that there are many people in the medical community that are quite aware that there are particular personality traits that are seen in people who have cancer.

In other words, the medical community knows that there are spiritual roots to disease. They know that certain thoughts, beliefs and behaviors are seen in people who have been diagnosed with cancer, and they know that these very issues can lead to cancer. However, we all know that doctors treat physical disease with physical solutions. They don't or rarely focus on the spiritual or emotional issues that can lead to a disease.

And what I have found is that this is the very place we have to investigate for healing.

Through the years, as I studied this issue, I found many doctors and researchers who were and are aware of this information and connection to the disease. I am going to present some of the information that has come out of these studies. My goal is to sift through the results of these studies and articles about them and relate them to God and His word.

Let's start by looking at an article about a study that is called, "Cancer Is A Message To You From Your Body[5]."

"Although choosing the right cancer treatment is important in your recovery, most only treat the physical symptom—the cancer itself— and completely overlook the underlying cause(s) of cancer.

Nearly all reported cases of cancer miracles documented report that the cancer survivor has made dramatic changes to their whole life. They have changed their diet and their lifestyle, they have removed all stress from their lives, and most importantly they have healed their internal emotional stress which is the primary cause of cancer.

Cancer is a physical symptom of prolonged internal emotional stress. Although most people endure stress and trauma during their life, it is the way we handle the stress—whether or not we repress our feelings and internalize the stress—that determines whether or not we get cancer. This may sound unreal to some. But, when you know how stress causes cancer, then and only then can you have the confidence to make the necessary changes and reverse cancer within your body.

Cancer is a message to you—from your body. It is communicating to you that something is not right within you—emotionally. Cancer is not a death sentence, it is an opportunity to heal within."

If you are truly looking to verify that there are spiritual and emotional roots to disease, I thought that the above was one of the most informative articles that I have read. The information that I was able to extrapolate from this study was that disease can be a message to you from your spirit and soul to your body. When we have symptoms or disease in our body, it is a message to us that something is not right in our lives.

In my own experience I have found that if I am entertaining negative beliefs, thinking, emotions and behaviors that don't line up with God and His word, my body can begin to have symptoms that can lead to and indicate that there is a disease process taking place.

Are You Thinking Like God?

If you understand God and His word and the concept of spiritual roots as found in "A More Excellent Way" by Dr. Henry Wright, the message is that your thinking is not in line with God.

The truth is that no disease has to be a death sentence. A disease can be viewed as just a way for you to see how your thoughts are affecting your body. If we know what thoughts and beliefs and behaviors that we are in agreement with that are leading to illness and disease, we can change them with God's help.

We know that if you have a disease or a symptom or an illness, that there can be a spiritual or an emotional root to the disease. Changing your spiritual or emotional condition can begin to change the chemistry in your body. When you change your chemistry, healing can happen.

Though these studies have information in them that can help us to see the underlying roots to these diseases, remember that these medical studies that I am presenting have nothing to do with God. They are not going to talk about remedies for the disease process of cancer that involve God or ministering His truth. But, the studies do show us that there is definitely a connection with how we think, believe and act and the health condition of our bodies.

Of course, Scripture tells us that too. I will present scriptures that support this after we look at the studies.

—— CHAPTER TWO ——

SCIENTIFIC STUDIES AND MEDICAL PROOF

A Cancer Personality

When I talk or minister to people who have been diagnosed with cancer, through the years, I have become aware of the thinking and behavioral issues that I see in the personality of a person who has the disease of cancer. I was seeing the same kinds of issues or personality traits in people who had cancer, so I began to research what the medical community has documented about the personality of the people who have cancer. I wanted some information from the medical community to support what I was seeing.

First, I will present several studies and articles about the studies, that were done about the types of thinking and behaviors that can be found in someone who has other disease processes besides cancer. These personality and behavior styles were studied by researchers to see what kinds of behaviors were associated with different diseases.

This will show you that researchers are aware that personality traits influence the disease processes that go on in our body. This is not only true for cancer, but it is true for more common diseases also. I want to present these articles and studies to you to verify that even the medical community knows that there are spiritual and emotional roots to diseases, in general.

Personality Type

This article shows the personality type and the disease process that can result.

"Your Personality Type Could Decide What Makes You Ill," by Roger Dobson[6]. These various personality types are:

Impulsive
You might expect impulsive types to be at risk from accidents but, in fact, their big health danger is stomach ulcers. Researchers at the Finnish Institute of Occupational Health studied more than 4,000 people and found that those who had an impulsive personality were 2.4 times more at risk for ulcers.

It's thought that impulsive people tend to respond to stress with higher than normal rates of acid production, triggering peptic ulcers. Research at the University of Wales has also shown that impulsiveness is associated with poorer control over eating.

Cheerful
One of the most surprising findings is that cheerful people are more likely to die early.

"Children who were rated by their parents and teachers as more cheerful, and as having a sense of humor, died earlier in adulthood than those who were less cheerful,' say University of California researchers. 'Contrary to expectation, cheerfulness and sense of humor were inversely related to longevity."

One theory is that cheerful people underestimate life's dangers and may also be more likely to have difficulty coping when things don't go as anticipated.

Anxious

People with anxiety disorders are three times more likely to be treated for high blood pressure. A study from Northern Arizona University found stress hormones may be the reason.

Meanwhile, women with phobic anxieties, such as fear of heights, were at higher risk of heart disease, high blood pressure and cholesterol. Although behavioral differences—like a greater tendency to smoke among people with anxiety—go some way to explaining why this happens, they do not explain it all.

Aggressive

Hostile types are prone to a range of serious health conditions, and there is plenty of research to back this up.

People who suffer from arthrosclerosis—furred up arteries—are more likely to have hostile personalities, according to a Scottish study based on almost 2,000 men and women.

An American study showed that aggressive types are at greater risk of chronic inflammation throughout the body, which is linked to a number of diseases including heart disease (inflammation is involved in the build-up of fatty deposits in the inner lining of the arteries). This could be because this personality type has higher levels of an immune system protein linked to inflammation.

Another theory is that hostile people respond more quickly and strongly to stress, both mentally and physiologically, increasing blood pressure and heart rate which results in more wear and tear on the cardiovascular system.

Angry types also take longer to heal. Researchers at Ohio State University created small wounds on the arms of healthy people, and after four days, only 30% of the angry patients' wounds had healed, compared to 70% of placid patients.

Aggressive types are also at higher risk for recurrent bouts of severe depression, according to another American study.

Shy

Socially inhibited people are more vulnerable to viral infections, suggests research from the University of California.

In animal studies, scientists found that gregarious types had more active protective lymph nodes than shy types. Lymph nodes are part of the body's immune system and help to destroy infectious germs, such as viruses like the common cold virus and bacteria.

Optimistic

People who always look on the bright side live an average of 7.5 years longer than those who take a gloomier view, according to work at the University of California.

And the risk of dying early from any disease is 55% lower for optimists, say researchers at

Wageningen University in the Netherlands who followed 1,000 people.

One theory is that optimism may increase the will to live, while another is that greater sociability plays a role; these in turn may lower levels of the stress hormone cortisol.

Researchers at Carnegie Mellon University in Pittsburgh[7] say that optimism boosts the immune system and protects from psychological stress. An American study showed that over a 30-year period, optimists had fewer disabilities and less chronic pain.

(My comment: This goes right along with God telling us to think on. Things that are of a good report!)

> Philippians 4:8 *Finally, brethren, whatsoever things are true, whatsoever things are honest, whatsoever things are just, whatsoever things are pure, whatsoever things are lovely, whatsoever things are of good report; if there be any virtue, and if there be any praise, think on these things.*

Tight-Lipped
Distressed types (also known as Type D personalities) suffer from a high degree of emotional suffering, but consciously suppress their feelings and as a result may be at higher risk of cancer and heart disease. Once Type D's develop coronary artery disease, they are at greater risk of dying, according to a Harvard University study.

The authors suggest that these people have poorly regulated stress hormones, meaning their hearts beat faster, blood pressure rises and blood vessels tighten—all bad for the cardiovascular system. Such types may also have more active immune systems, and therefore more inflammation, which results in damage to blood vessels.

Conscientious

This is the personality trait most associated with long life, according to a University of California study. It has as significant an effect on longevity as maintaining healthy blood pressure and cholesterol levels, research from Nottingham University suggests. Thought conscientious people avoid risk and are more likely to adopt and maintain healthy behaviors.

Neurotic

If being a neurotic type wasn't hard work enough, it's also associated with asthma, headaches, stomach ulcers and heart disease, according to a University of California study.

It's suggested that neurotic types often employ less effective coping strategies, with lots of self blame and hostility, rather than seeking help and support. They therefore may become more stressed, resulting in a less effective immune system and greater vulnerability to disease. Another theory is that neurotics are more likely to be depressed, and depression lowers the immune system.

Extrovert

Like optimists, they are less likely to get heart disease, according to a Milan University study.

Italian researchers found that the biggest extroverts were 15 percent less likely to get disease. They are also more likely to recover quickly from disease, and less prone to infections.

One theory is that they have more effective coping strategies so fewer stress hormones. They may also be more likely to seek medical help for symptoms. But one downside is that, according to research at Yamagata University School of Medicine in Japan, they are more likely to be obese than neurotics. Theories range from behavioral differences, with extroverts more likely to be sociable and therefore eat more.

Pessimistic

Those who always expect the worst will find that when it comes to health, they're right: pessimists have a 19 percent increased risk of dying early compared to optimists.

Researchers in America have also found that people who have high levels of pessimism and anxiety have an increased risk of developing Parkinson's disease decades later.

"What we have shown for the first time is that there's a link between an anxious or pessimistic personality and the future development of Parkinson's," says neurologist Dr. James Bower from the Mayo Clinic. "What we didn't find is the explanation for that link. It remains unclear whether anxiety and pessimism are risk factors for Parkinson's disease, or are linked to Parkinson's disease via common risk factors or a common genetic predisposition."

These studies give us a look into the kinds of studies that the medical community has done on diseases other than cancer. They show us the connections between certain ways of thinking and the disease consequences that can be associated with them.

Cancer and Personality

Let's go on and begin to look at the studies and articles that refer to cancer, starting with this article on "Personality Types and Cancer:"

Lawrence LeShan, MD[8], was one of the early figures introducing what has become a renaissance of these ideas. In the sixties, LeShan suggested that cancer was more prevalent in certain personality types. He described what became known as the carcinogenic personality— someone who began life feeling deprived or incomplete and powerless to do anything about it. As an adult, this personality appears to fill the perceived emptiness with another person, or external object, which affords them a sense of belonging, status, or power. The cancer patients LeShan studied had experienced a loss of this external source of "wholeness" within the previous six months due to a death, retirement, loss of job, etc.

The evidence has accumulated steadily, indicating that our state of mind impacts our health, with the nervous and immune systems serving as mediators.

[Since most of us are co-dependent, you might think we are all cancer-prone, but our choice of diseases seems to depend on our style of attempting to fill our perceived internal void (fostered by our culture of estrangement).

Cancer-prone individuals seem to go about it more passively than the Type A personality most frequently associated with heart disease. Both are different external defenses against the primal feeling of incompleteness.]

Here is more information in this article about this study:

Is there such a thing as a "cancer personality?" A 1984 study measured the physiological responses to stressful stimuli of three groups: patients with malignant melanoma (a potentially fatal form of skin cancer), people with heart disease, and a control cohort with no medical illness.

This study demonstrated that people can experience emotional stresses with measurable physical effects on their system—while managing to sequester their feelings in a place completely beyond conscious awareness.

It was in relationship to melanoma that the notion of a Type C personality was first proposed, a combination of emotional traits more likely to be found in those who develop cancer than in people who remain free of it. Type C personalities have been described as extremely cooperative, patient, passive, accepting, and lacking assertiveness.

The characteristics associated with the Type C

personality all represent emotional repression, a pushing down of necessary emotions. In contrast, self-assertion is important to having our needs met. Avoiding conflict and wanting to be liked lead to the denial of these needs.

Thus the repression of emotions threatens not only our psychological health but also our physical well-being. It does so by suppressing our immune response. In turn, immune suppression leaves us susceptible to bacterial or viral invaders [e.g. Cancer], or to malignant changes from within.

First, note that the personality type for cancer is referred to as Type C. I also want to point out the personality styles that are mentioned here. Type C personalities have been described as extremely cooperative, patient, passive, accepting, and lacking assertiveness. The characteristics associated with the Type C personality all represent emotional repression, a pushing down of necessary emotions.

The important issue here is—are you telling the truth about how you really think and feel? Are you fabricating your personality? Do you tell the truth to yourself, God and others?

We are going to explore these issues in more depth later in this book.

Cancer From Unresolved Conflicts

To continue, let's look at some other articles and studies that have to do with cancer.

Dr. Ryke-Geerd Hamer's German New Medicine[8]

Cancer surgeon Dr. Ryke-Geerd Hamer from
Germany has examined 20,000 cancer patients
with all types of cancer. Dr. Hamer noticed that
all his patients seemed to have something in
common: there had been some kind of psycho-
emotional conflict prior to the onset of their
cancer—usually a few years before—a conflict
that had never fully resolved. Dr. Hamer started
including psychotherapy as an important part
of the healing process and found that when
the specific conflict was resolved, the cancer
immediately stopped growing at a cellular level.
Dr. Hamer believes that cancer people are unable
to share their thoughts, emotions, fears and
joys with other people. He calls this "psycho-
emotional isolation." These people tend to hide
away sadness and grief behind a brave face,
appear 'nice' and avoid open conflict. Some
are not even aware of their emotions, and are
therefore not only isolated from other people, but
also from themselves.

This cancer researcher, Dr. Hamer, has found
that people with cancer have had a trauma before
the cancer diagnosis. He also noticed that it was
not the trauma that caused the body to have an
environment that allowed cancer to grow. Dr.
Hamer said that it was how the person handled the
trauma that was the thing that set the person up
for either being healthy or having a disease process.
He related that if the conflict was not resolved, the
people were more likely to have an environment in
their body that supports cancer. He said that the
people did not share their feelings, that they were
actually putting on a brave face, they appeared

nice, but, they were essentially in denial and they avoided the conflict and their feelings."

Sometimes we don't even know that we are in denial. We are just trying to deal with something that caused us pain, and we don't have the Godly skills to deal with the issues that can happen to us in life.

In order to come to a place of peace with ourselves, with God and with other people, we have to work out our traumas with God.

Here is more information from this same study by Dr. Hamer:

Dr. Hamer has come up with some revolutionary information. X-rays taken of the brain by Dr. Hamer showed in all cases a 'dark shadow' somewhere in the brain. These dark spots would be in exactly the same place in the brain for the same types of cancer. There was also a 100% correlation between the dark spot in the brain, the location of the cancer in the body and the specific type of unresolved conflict.

On the basis of these findings, Dr. Hamer suggests that when we are in a stressful conflict that is not resolved, the emotional reflex center in the brain which corresponds to the experienced emotion (e.g: anger, frustration, grief) will slowly break down. Each of these emotion centers are connected to a specific organ. When a center breaks down, it will start sending wrong information to the organ it controls, resulting in the formation of deformed cells in the tissues: cancer cells. He also suggests that metastases are not the SAME cancer spreading. It is the result of new conflicts that may well be brought on by the very stress of having cancer or of invasive and painful or nauseating therapies.

This part of the article about the doctor's observations suggest that unresolved conflicts can affect us and our propensity towards disease. It also suggests why one part of our bodies may be affected by disease, as opposed to another part of our bodies. Dr. Hamer says that it is the kind of conflict that relates to different parts of our brains that determines what part of our bodies will be affected.

The Cancer Personality

Let's continue to look at "The Cancer Personality" by Gabor Mate, M.D[9].

Is there such a thing as a "cancer personality"? A 1984 study measured the physiological responses to stressful stimuli of three groups: patients with malignant melanoma (a potentially fatal form of skin cancer), people with heart disease, and a control cohort with no medical illness. Each person was connected to a dermograph, a device that recorded the body's electrical reactions in the skin as the subject looked at a series of slides designed to elicit psychological distress. The slides displayed unpleasant statements such as "You're ugly" or "You have only yourself to blame."

Participants were asked to record their subjective awareness of how disturbed they felt on reading each statement and their physiological responses were registered. The researchers thus secured a printout of the actual level of nervous system distress each participant experienced. They also secured a simultaneous report of the subject's conscious perception of emotional stress.

Although physiological responses among the three groups were identical, the melanoma group proved most likely to deny any awareness that the messages on the slides upset them emotionally. This study demonstrated that people can experience emotional stresses with measurable physical effects on their system—while managing to sequester their feelings in a place completely beyond conscious awareness.

It was in relationship to melanoma that the notion of a Type C personality was first proposed, a combination of emotional traits more likely to be found in those who develop cancer than in people who remain free of it. Type C personalities have been described as extremely cooperative, patient, passive, accepting, and lacking assertiveness.

These same traits have now been found in studies of many other cancers as well. In 1991, researchers in Melbourne, Australia, investigated whether personality traits were a risk factor in cancer of the colon. Over 600 people, newly diagnosed, were compared with a matched group of controls. Cancer patients, to a statistically significant degree, were more likely to demonstrate elements of denial and repression of anger. They appeared to be "nice" people who suppressed reactions to avoid conflict.

The characteristics associated with the Type C personality all represent emotional repression, a pushing down of necessary emotions. In contrast, self-assertion is important to having our needs met. Avoiding conflict and wanting to be liked lead to the denial of these needs.

How do emotional traits translate into cancerous skin lesions or other malignancies? The answer is that biology and psychology are not independent; each represents the functioning of a super system with components that can no longer be thought of as separate or autonomous mechanisms. The past quarter century of scientific inquiry has supplanted the traditional Western medical view of a split between body and mind with a truer, more unitary perspective. Our mind and body are one and our physiology, including our immune system, is directly affected by our emotions.

Thus the repression of emotions threatens not only our psychological health but also our physical well-being. It does so by suppressing our immune response. In turn, immune suppression leaves us susceptible to bacterial or viral invaders [e.g. Cancer], or to malignant changes from within.

How Are You Reacting?

This information also tells us that according to the kind of conflict or trauma that we have had and how we feel and think about that trauma, different parts of our brain will be affected and this can determine what kind of cancer the person may present.

In other words, how are you reacting to the traumatic event that has occurred in your life?

What we learn here is this: How you deal with the issues in your life can determine how healthy your body is. This information supports what we know about our thoughts, beliefs, attitudes and behaviors and how they can become roots to diseases that manifest in our bodies.

Cancer Cells

Biologically, in very basic terms, cancer cells are healthy cells gone "bad." They have formed a defect or mutation of some kind. They do not follow "rules" as normal cells do and totally disregard them. Normal healthy cells grow and divide and function the way they were designed to function; when old cells "wear-out" and die, new ones divide and form. It's a balanced system. They receive normal regulating cell cycle signals when the proper environment and nutrients are present for the cell to grow.

Cancer cells grow and divide with complete disregard for this balanced system; complete disregard for the needs and limitations of the body. They are aggressive and destructive. Cancer cells are not able to receive normal signals that regulate the normal cell cycle. Cancer cells also do not stop dividing even when nutrients and growth factors are depleted. However, cancer cells do require nutrients to grow, but they steal them from the surrounding healthy tissue.

Normal cells stop dividing when they receive

signals that a nutrient is depleted, or the environment is not conducive to growth. Normal cells also stay in the general place in the body they were formed and designed to stay---example, skin cells continue to grow new skin, they don't move on to the muscle and begin producing muscle cells. Cancer cells can and do move to other parts of the body; they spread.

This study supports the concept of roots to disease that we see in "A More Excellent Way" by Dr. Henry Wright. He says that there are specific roots to specific diseases. He has named many of these roots in this book and in his ministry.

I present another study to help us understand this concept.

Scientists from Cancer Research UK[10] have taken advantage of the selfish behavior of cancer cells to target them with a genetically engineered virus. If infected by a virus, normal cells altruistically shut themselves down to contain the virus, but cancer cells refuse to stop for anything—allowing the virus to thrive. Researchers found it was able to spread throughout tumors, leaving healthy tissue untouched.

When I read this I saw that one characteristic of cancer cells is that they are selfish.

Cancer cells themselves, are selfish!

This was so interesting to me, because it supports the fact that your body will conform to the thoughts and beliefs that you allow to stay in your mind. Your body will conform to whatever you think and believe to be true. Your body conforms to your thoughts.

Following this train of thought and this logic, the truth is that your cells in your body are conforming to what you believe to be true. Your cells in your body will conform to your thoughts and attitudes. So if cancer cells are selfish, self-focused and self-serving, and your cells are conforming to your thoughts, beliefs and attitudes, then you might extrapolate from that information that your thoughts, beliefs and attitudes might be selfish.

What is my point? People with cancer can have as their thoughts, beliefs and attitudes, a personality pattern of being selfish, self-centered, self-focused and narcissistic. They can also be in agreement with a spirit of self-pity. They think that everything is about them. They have their minds on themselves. This can be idolatry to the self.

This truth that cancer cells are selfish is a truth that I find to be true in the person's personality when I talk to and minister to people who have cancer.

You might ask, "Isn't everyone selfish?" The answer is that we are all concerned about taking care of ourselves, but I am talking about a self-focus that is very profound. It is a self-focus that often comes out of fear and the need to keep ourselves safe. It also has a sense of entitlement that things should go our way, and if they don't we can become very disappointed. Disappointment leads directly to anger. Instead of being flexible the person holds onto the regret and the anger and the disappointment that they felt. They do not work this out with God. The problem is not that we become angry; the problem is that we don't work out our anger in a healthy and Godly way.

Being angry is not the problem, but how you handle and work out your anger is going to make all of the difference in your life. The Bible tells us this in:

Ephesians 4:26 *Be ye angry, and sin not.*

We are going to be angry, but we don't want to sin in our anger. Some examples of sinful reactions to anger may be yelling, screaming, retaliation, silent treatments, holding a grudge, gossiping, hitting, and throwing things or anything that does not line up with Godly behaviors.

Things will happen while we are on this planet that will cause us to be angry. We don't live in a perfect world. We have to know and understand that God never promises us that we will get everything we want or that nothing negative will happen to us. On the contrary, He tells us this:

Matthew 5:45 *That ye may be the children of your Father which is in heaven: for he maketh his sun to rise on the evil and on the good, and sendeth rain on the just and on the unjust.*

Jesus came to tell us that even though we are all subject to the problems and tribulations in the world, when we believe in Him and choose Him as our Savior, He will help us to overcome the problems that we encounter in the world.

John 16:33 *These things I have spoken unto you, that in me ye might have peace. In the world ye shall have tribulation: but be of good cheer; I have overcome the world.*

A Life Changing Truth

The truth is that all of us are going to have problems while we are on this planet. It is how we deal with the problems that will determine our emotional, physical and spiritual health.

While we are alive on this planet, we can always change the way that we think and believe and behave. And, God can help us do just that!

Philippians 2:12 *Wherefore, my beloved, as ye have always obeyed, not as in my presence only, but now much more in my absence, work out your own salvation with fear and trembling.*

Every day of our lives brings us an opportunity to work with God to confess and repent for our thoughts, beliefs and behaviors that don't line up with His. I call the next part of our work with God, "The Great Exchange." We have to exchange our old thoughts and beliefs and behaviors with the new ones that we learn that come from God and His word, the Bible.

One more important point that I would like to make is that I know for sure that what we think will influence the health of our bodies. A scripture that supports this view is this:

Proverbs 23:7 *For as he thinketh in his heart, so is he.*

As you think in your heart, what you think about and what you believe to be true—so you will have the opportunity to be. What you think and what you believe will have the opportunity to determine who you are.

Going back to the last article: if you are selfish, your body may conform to that reality, and allow selfish cancer cells to thrive. Remember, the Bible tells us that what you think you are and you can become.

Here is another study that says just this, it is called:

The Nocebo Effect: Placebo's Evil Twin, B. Brian Reid[11]

Special to The Washington Post
Tuesday, April 30, 2002; Page HE01

Ten years ago, researchers stumbled onto a striking finding: Women who believed that they were prone to heart disease were nearly four times as likely to die as women with similar risk factors who didn't hold such fatalistic views.

The higher risk of death, in other words, had nothing to with the usual heart disease culprits— age, blood pressure, cholesterol, weight, instead it tracked closely with belief. Think sick, be sick.

That study is a classic in the annals of research on the "nocebo" phenomenon, the evil twin of the placebo effect. While the placebo effect refers to health benefits produced by a treatment that should have no effect, patients experiencing the nocebo effect experience the opposite. "They presume the worst, health-wise, and that's just what they get. They're convinced that something is going to go wrong, and it's a self-fulfilling prophecy," said Arthur Barsky, a psychiatrist at Boston's Brigham and Women's Hospital who published an article earlier this year in the Journal of the American Medical Association beseeching his peers to pay closer attention to the nocebo effect. "From a clinical point of view, this is by no means peripheral or irrelevant."

Think Sick, Be Sick

The comment in the article that impacted me most was, "think sick, be sick."

What you think is what you become. If you think that you are sick, you are more likely to be sick. What you say with your mouth is how you really think and feel.

God is really smart, He made sure that He put Proverbs 23:7 in the Bible: *What a man thinks in his heart, so is he.*

What we think and say about ourselves and the world is what we can become.

I found another article that I thought was interesting and goes right along with what scripture says.

"Positive feelings may be key to effective cancer cure[12]"

Scientists say they have found that one of the body's "good mood chemicals" forces some cancer cells to commit suicide. They say that when serotonin is placed in a test tube alongside tumor cells of Burkitt's lymphoma the cancer kills itself. The scientists from the University of Birmingham add that when the chemical is produced by the body it prevents depression. Quote: "An exciting property of serotonin is that it can tell some cells to self-destruct. We have found serotonin can get inside the lymphoma cells and instruct them to commit suicide."

We can extrapolate from this that if we change our thoughts and our moods we can raise our serotonin. Raising our serotonin can promote healing in our bodies and minds.

God's Thinking

What this is telling us is just what God tells us in Scripture.

2 Corinthians 10:5 *Casting down imaginations, and every high thing that exalteth itself against the knowledge of God, and bringing into captivity every thought to the obedience of Christ;*

Philippians 4:8 *Finally, brethren, whatsoever things are true, whatsoever things are honest, whatsoever things are just, whatsoever things are pure, whatsoever things are lovely, whatsoever things are of good report; if there be any virtue, and if there be any praise, think on these things.*

We are told by God to think about Godly things and cast down imaginations or thoughts or beliefs or ideas, that don't agree with God and His word. This is not what the world calls positive thinking, it is something that I call GOD'S THINKING.

Positive thinking is just putting thoughts in your mind that you or the world sees as being positive. They may or may not line up with God and His word. God's thinking includes thoughts and beliefs that line up with the truth that God tells us in the Bible. It is what our creator tells us is true.

An example: A person thinks "I am going to get drunk tonight so that I feel better." That may feel like positive thinking to the individual, but in reality it is destructive and not healthy. Our goal is to think Godly thoughts! Godly thoughts lead us into all truth and ultimately health.

Here is an article on Developing and Healing Cancer:

The Power of Thought to Make Ill and Heal[13], by thinking about good things (*or godly things*):

Some of the most valuable work has been done by Dr. Caroline Bedell Thomas of Johns Hopkins University Medical School. Beginning in 1946, she took personality profiles of 1,337 medical students, then surveyed their mental and physical health every year for decades after graduation. Her goal was to find psychological antecedents of heart disease, high blood pressure, mental illness, and suicide.

She included cancer in the study for the sake of comparison, because she originally thought it would have no psychological component.

However, the data showed a "striking and unexpected" result: the traits of those who developed cancer were almost identical to those of the students who later committed suicide. Almost all the cancer patients had throughout their lives been restricted in expressing emotion, especially aggressive emotions related to their own needs. She also found that, using only the drawings they made as one of the tests, she could predict what parts of their bodies would develop cancer."

In his conversations with Bill Moyers, Michael Lerner, co-founder of the Commonwealth Cancer Help Program, cites a study by Lydia Temoshek, whose work was also cited by Cousins of patients with malignant melanoma: "Temoshek looked at the difference between patients who expressed their feelings and those who didn't, and discovered that the ones who expressed their feelings had more immune activity at the site of their lesions. They also had thinner lesions than the people who did not express their feelings."

Expressing Feelings

One of the most prevalent personality traits that I see and read about in someone who has cancer is that they do not express their feelings.

Sometimes I have heard people say that feelings are devils and you can just cast them out. I have heard people say, "Do you want to have feelings, or do you want to be like Jesus?" What we have to remember is that feelings are just feelings.

Jesus had feelings and He expressed His feelings.

The shortest scripture in the Bible shows us Jesus expressing and feeling His feelings.

John 11:35 *Jesus wept.*

We are created in God's image and He has feelings. Something else that we have to know is that feelings can be liars. Feelings are not emergencies. We don't have to do what our feelings tell us and we don't have to be in agreement with what our feelings tell us. However, we do have to acknowledge what we are feeling and decide to deal with our feelings and emotions in a Godly way.

We have to learn to cast down our thoughts, cast out devils and deal with our feelings in a Godly way. A lot of the time we are not taught how to identify and express our feelings in healthy ways. One of the most important things that we have to learn about is how to deal with our feelings. Sometimes people don't even know what it is that they are feeling. It is important for us to acknowledge our feelings and then deal with them with God in a Godly way.

To learn a lot more about this subject of "feeling your feelings," please see my booklet called "Freedom to Feel[2]"

Here is an article that talks about the tendency for the cancer patient to NOT express their feelings.

One of the best-known mental predictors of cancer is the "cancer personality type[14]." Cousins sites the work of psychologist Lawrence LeShan, an early pioneer in this field: LeShan—research psychologist of the Institute of Applied Biology in New York—conducted extensive pioneering work regarding the cancer-prone personality that led him to identify several psychological characteristics that seemed to typify cancer patients (including such factors as the inability to express aggression and disruption of a parental relationship in early childhood). He concluded that personality factors have some bearing on the observed association between traumatic life events (most notably, the loss of a significant emotional relationship) and the development of cancer, and he speculated that specific psychological attributes could be linked to particular types and locations of cancer. **One of the more important traits of the cancer personality type is an inability to express emotions.** Siegel, who calls it an inability to "be your own person," says:" As Elida Evans observed in her ground-breaking 1926 study of the cancer personality, 'Development of individuality is a safeguard to life and health.'"

Let's look at another article that I think is interesting. It has to do with cancer personality styles.

Personality and Cancer—How Personality Impacts Health Oct. 21, 2007, Christine Scivicque[15]

Recent studies show that certain personality types are more likely to be diagnosed with Cancer than others. Discover the common personality traits and the reasons why.

Most people are familiar with the idea of the "Heart Attack Personality" ("Type A": hostile, aggressive, prone to emotional outbursts).

However, few people are aware that there is also a typical "Cancer Personality" as well. The common character traits shared by cancer patients have been studied and documented in recent years, and now many holistic practitioners are addressing these issues as a part of the healing process.

It is important to recognize that everyone has cancer cells in their body. We have trillions of cells in our bodies and there is an ongoing process in which millions of cells die and millions of others divide to replace them. During this process, the DNA sequence is passed along from one cell to another. A cancer cell develops when the sequence is modified or mutated during the division process. This may happen for a variety of reasons, including viruses, bacteria or parasites, nuclear or electromagnetic radiation, chemical exposure, free radicals or aging DNA. Research shows that a healthy person may have around 10,000 cancer cells in their body at any given time. Typically, the immune system destroys the cancer cells before they can divide and form new ones.

Cancer tumors develop in weakened or traumatized parts of the body. What weakens the body and the immune system's ability to destroy the cancer cells? Studies show that one's personality plays a large role in this. Researchers believe individuals fitting the "Type C" personality are at greater risk for developing cancer.

Several traits define this personality type:

- Poor ability to cope with stress
- Highly conscientious, responsible and caring (particularly for others): These individuals often have a tendency to take on the burdens of others.
- Deep desire to make others happy, often at their own expense (people pleasers)
- Harboring suppressed toxic emotions (anger, resentment or hostility): These individuals often show an inability to express and resolve deep emotional problems or conflicts and are often unaware of their presence.
- History of lack of closeness with one or both parents, perhaps resulting in the same lack of closeness with a spouse.

This research is strong evidence of the mind-body connection, proving that the health of the mind deeply impacts that of the body. Ongoing suppression and internalization of emotion weakens the body. However, many argue that personality directly influences behavior. Those matching the above personality traits may be more likely to engage in unhealthy behaviors, such as smoking. Whatever the reason, the correlation suggests that managing these "personality traits" may be a necessary step towards recovery.

Making some minor lifestyle adjustments, such as managing stress and improving diet, can have a significant impact on health.

It is important for people to be aware that their mental state, their behaviors and reactions to the world around them, and their strategies for dealing with emotions are an important part of being healthy. Running a mile a day and taking vitamins won't counteract the effects of what goes on internally. Self-awareness and continual self-improvement have a critical role in healing and preventing disease.

Please review the traits that define this personality type. Can you relate to any of these personality traits?

If you do, this is a great time to begin to recognize these traits and purpose in your heart to exchange them with traits that line up with God and His word. We want to exchange the traits that can lead to sickness and disease with traits that lead to being healthy.

We can admit our sins, quit our sins and exchange them with the ways of God. We can go to God and confess and repent for our sins.

1 John 1:9 *If we confess our sins, he is faithful and just to forgive us our sins, and to cleanse us from all unrighteousness.*

This is the beginning of our change and transformation into the image of Jesus Christ. We can see that the medical community knows that our personality—or what we think and believe and do—can create an environment in our bodies to be susceptible to cancer.

When we begin to recognize and change our thoughts and behaviors so that they line up with God and His word and ways, our bodies and lives can be healed.

The loaded statement from the previous article quotation is, "Individuals fitting the Type C personality are at a greater risk for developing cancer."

That is the main point of all of this information. These ways of thinking and behaving can open you up to having an environment in your body that can be conducive to supporting the disease of cancer. The medical community knows this information.

Are You a Type C (Cancer) Personality? By Dr. Jean-Jacques Dugoua, M.D.[16]

According to behavioral oncologists, the façade of pleasantness with a Type C personality will collapse over time due to the impact of accumulated stressors, especially those evoking feelings of depression and reactions of helplessness and hopelessness. The coping style of Type C personalities, i.e. excessive denial, avoidance, suppression and repression of emotions, appears to weaken natural resistance to carcinogenic influences.

Recent studies show that psycho-social stressors which are characterized by inadequate and repressive coping mechanisms are associated with changes in immune competency, including both humoral and cell-mediated immunity. Relationships between different immune parameters (natural killer cell activity, lymphocytes, serotonin uptake, mean platelet volume) and mood states, psychological coping styles and personality variables have been discovered.

Deny, Avoid, Suppress, Repress or Ignore

This study is so important to understand. When people deny, ignore, avoid, suppress and repress their emotions, it weakens their immune system.

I want to make sure that you understand what each of these terms mean:

Deny: *To refuse to recognize or acknowledge or to state that (something declared or believed to be true) is not true.* This means that we just don't face something at all, we are in denial as if the issue just does not exist.

Avoid: *To keep away from; keep clear of; to shun.* This means that we just don't deal with the issue. We avoid it at all costs.

Ignore: *To not acknowledge.* It means that it does not even exist. It is as if you had a big pink elephant in your living room and you ignore it. You just keep watching TV as if it were not even there.

Suppress: *To put an end to forcibly; to subdue. To curtail or prohibit the activities of. To keep from being revealed, published, or circulated. To deliberately exclude (unacceptable desires or thoughts) from the mind. To inhibit the expression of (an impulse, for example); check: suppress a smile.* This means that we just won't allow ourselves to talk about or deal with an issue even though we know it is there. If a controversial issue pops into our mind, we just push it down or subdue it again.

Repress: *1. To keep under control, check, or suppress (desires, feelings, actions, tears, etc.). 2.*

To keep down or suppress (anything objectionable).
3. To put down or quell (sedition, disorder, etc.). 4.
To reduce (persons) to subjection. 5. Psychoanalysis.
To reject (painful or disagreeable ideas, memories,
feelings, or impulses) from the conscious mind.

This means when we don't deal with the issues in our lives in a Godly way, we may be engaging in one of these personality styles that can eventually be conducive to disease.

Michael Jawer in the book he wrote with Marc Micozzi, M.D, Ph.D., called" The Spiritual Anatomy of Emotion: How Feelings Link the brain, the Body and the Sixth Sense," discusses the new Type C Personality. Here is a brief excerpt of their description of that personality type:

In recent years, a cluster of personality characteristics has come to be identified as the Type C personality, someone who is at heightened risk for a slew of afflictions, from colds to asthma to cancer. In contrast with the Type A person (who angers easily and has difficulty keeping feelings under wraps) and the Type B person (who has a healthier balance of emotional expressiveness), the Type C person is a suppressor, a stoic, a denier of feelings. He or she has a calm, outwardly rational, and unemotional demeanor, but also a tendency to conform to the wishes of others, a lack of assertiveness, and an inclination toward feelings of helplessness or hopelessness.

This is the sort of personality that Canadian physician Gabor Mate has studied extensively.

Over his years of family practice, Mate relates, he began to notice a pattern: individuals who were unable to express anger, who didn't seem to recognize the primacy of their own needs, and who were constantly doing for others, appeared to be the ones most susceptible to a slew of ailments, from asthma, rheumatoid arthritis, and lupus to multiple sclerosis and amyotrophic lateral sclerosis. These conditions are all autoimmune disorders. Mate claims that, when an individual engages in a long-term practice of ignoring or suppressing legitimate feelings–when he or she is just plain too nice–the immune system can become compromised and confused, learning to attack the self rather than defend it.

Emotional expression, in Mate's view is absolutely essential because feelings serve to alert the individual to what is dangerous or unwholesome–or, conversely, to what is helpful and nourishing–so that the person can either take protective action against the thread or move toward the beneficial stimulus. If someone never gets angry, this reflects an unhealthy inability or unwillingness to defend personal integrity. Such "boundary confusion" can ultimately become a matter of life and death. If someone just cannot say no, Mate argues, his or her body will end up saying it in the form of illness or disease.

I want to make sure that you read this again that the Type C person is a suppressor, a stoic, a denier of feelings. He or she has a calm, outwardly rational, and unemotional demeanor, but also a tendency to conform to the wishes of others, a lack of assertiveness, and an inclination toward feelings of helplessness or hopelessness. (As presented in "Mediation Matters", a blog by Steve Mehta.[17]

Do you recognize any of these traits in your own personality? Recognition is the first step to change and transformation.

I thought that this was so interesting. This article acknowledges how important it is for us to acknowledge understand our feelings. It also acknowledges how important it is to know what we are feeling. But, the thing that interests me the most is that the writer acknowledges that we know that feelings are just feelings. We check them out and then decide what to do with them.

We should do what the Scripture says, be angry and sin not.

Ephesians 4:26 *Be ye angry, and sin not: let not the sun go down upon your wrath:*

Acknowledge and Deal with Feelings

We can extrapolate from this scripture that it does not matter what feelings we have. We can have our feelings, for example: we can be angry, we can be sad, but we don't sin because we are angry or sad. We can be embarrassed but we sin not. We can be disappointed and still decide to sin not. We can have feelings. It is okay to have feelings, we just don't want to sin because of the feelings that we have.

Feelings are just feelings, they are the results of our experiences and how we react to these experiences. Remember that feelings are not emergencies. Just because we have a feeling, we don't have to act on that feeling, but we should acknowledge it, confess it and check it out with God. We should then be able to deal with the feeling in a Godly way.

We have to learn to know what we are feeling and thinking. We can't just let our minds be a waste dump of thoughts and emotions. We have to watch our thoughts that lead to our feelings and that eventually lead to our beliefs and behaviors.

In all of these cases, if we are listening to the devil and not dealing with our issues with God and in a Godly way, we may be setting ourselves up for potential problems in our lives. It is important to remember that we should be thinking and behaving in Godly ways in order to have a healthy body, spirit and soul.

Again, remember, personality styles, characteristics of thinking and behaving can and do have an effect on your health.

Here is a comment from one of the articles that I read about studies that help us to understand more about our feelings and how they relate to our health:

In sum, the studies indicate that despair, a profound feeling of sadness coupled with a sense of resignation to conditions, is the attitude that is least healthy when attempting to recover from cancer. Secondly, the social style of not expressing one's negative emotions, especially if it stems from an exaggerated fear of others disapproval, seems to describe the personality profile of those most likely to get cancer in the first place[13].

If we are hopeless and don't have hope for change for the future, this is not good for our immune system function. If we are fabricating our personality to please others to avoid conflict, fear or rejection, this is also not good for a strong immune system.

Let's continue to look at the personality traits that seem to accompany cancer and we will sift everything through God and His word.

Personality Traits

I want to present another article called Simran Healing[18], that I read that I think is important.

[Not the source of this quote]
"To many, a disease comes as a surprise. A sudden heart attack or gall stones or cancer diagnosis do shock them and they keep recounting how they were living a healthy life with not even a fever or cold. They keep asking their Doctor about the cause. The answers given, range from blame being given to viruses, food, stress or their life style. The fact, however, is different. The cause is internal and the starting point is "how they think and behave."

Today, research in mind-body connection clearly points that mind influences the body towards both health and disease. Anger, guilt, jealousy, anxiety, victim mentality, grief, remorse and other multitude of mind states influence negatively our body's physiology on a daily basis whereas the positive state of mind comprising love, warmth, confidence, helpfulness, etc. keep our body healthy.

Below lists some examples of diseases linked with mind-states by medical researchers:

Anger, hostile behavior and depressive symptoms in apparently healthy individuals may lead to cardiovascular disease and stroke - Psychosomatic Medicine (September 2004)

Anxiety disorders have been linked with Oral health problems - General Dentistry (November/ December 2003)

People who are happy and relaxed may have more Immunity to Common Cold than those who are depressed, nervous or angry - Psychosomatic Medicine (July 2003)

Angry resentment has been related to functional gastric complaints, particularly where patients reported unfair treatment in a study by IRVING D. HARRIS, MAJOR, MEDICAL CORPS, A.U.S - Psychosomatic Medicine

Clinically, allergic children have been found to suffer from Maternal Rejection in a study by Hyman Miller M.D. and Dorothy W. Buruch Ph.D. University of Southern California Medical School and reported in - Psychosomatic Medicine

All of this information points to the fact that what we think and believe and how we behave can be responsible for the health of our bodies.

The Personality - Mind-Body Connection

This is an article by the Deborah King Center[19] worth mentioning: "A sad soul can kill you quicker than a germ" - John Steinbeck

"There has been no direct link discovered between stress and the development of cancer, but in my healing work with thousands of individuals, I have seen that link. Here's how it happens: when children develop the habit of holding in their emotions, a traumatic event as an adult—like a car accident or divorce—can be the straw that breaks the camel's back of your health. Anything that makes us feel that we don't have control over our life can throw us totally sideways. A personal tragedy may result in an excess level of stress, which can create immune deficiency. Combined with underlying personality traits and a habit of suppressing emotion, cells can start proliferating in an unhealthy way. Western Medicine requires visible proof, so they haven't seen a link since it is difficult to quantitatively measure stress. It is also impossible to separate stress from behaviors caused by stress, such as drinking, smoking, eating poorly, and more. These factors can cause cancer too. Cancer is not just a physical disease. It is a disease of the mind and soul as much as it is of the body."

The last line in this article is very profound. Cancer is a disease that manifests in our physical body, but it has spiritual roots in our soul and our spirit.

Our immune system is affected by our thoughts. A compromised immune system can be the very reason that we have a disease process in our bodies. When we have had a rough childhood, very often that can set us up for a compromised immune system.

The Effect of Childhood Trauma on Brain Development

As recently as the 1980s, many professionals thought that by the time babies are born, the structure of their brains was already genetically determined. However, emerging research shows evidence of altered brain functioning as a result of early abuse and neglect[20].

Here is another article that connects childhood trauma and cancer:

The relationship between self-reported childhood trauma and the presence of a diagnosis of cancer during adult life was examined in the present study. Data were taken from the 1994/95 Canadian National Population Health Survey[21] of 15,106 Canadians. Childhood trauma, was measured by a 7-item index (reflecting physical abuse, fearful experiences, being sent away from home, hospitalization and parental disturbance). The presence of trauma during childhood was associated with higher cancer rates during adulthood, and each increase in the types of trauma that were experienced was associated with an increase in cancer (see graph). For example, those who were exposed to three or more types of trauma had more than twice the odds of a cancer diagnosis than those who reported no trauma.

Here is another article that talks about a study that relates childhood trauma to cancer:

Will Childhood Trauma Lead to Lung Cancer[22]?

(Ivanhoe Newswire) - Adverse events in childhood have been linked to an increase in the likelihood of developing lung cancer later in life. The link is partly explained by raised rates of cigarette smoking in victims of childhood trauma, but researchers note that other factors also may be to blame. David Brown and Robert Anda from the Centers for Disease Control and Prevention, worked with a team of researchers to study the effects of emotional, physical and sexual abuse, witnessing domestic violence, parental separation, or growing up in a household where people were mentally ill, substance abusers, or sent to prison. "Adverse childhood experiences were associated with an increased risk of lung cancer," Brown was quoted as saying, "particularly premature death from lung cancer. Although smoking behaviors, including early smoking initiation and heavy smoking, account for the greater part of this risk, other mechanisms or pathophysiologic pathways may be involved."

Adverse event information was collected from 17,337 people between 1995 and 1997. Brown and colleagues followed up on the medical records of these same people to study lung cancer rates in 2005.

"Compared to those who claimed no childhood trauma, people who experienced six or more traumas were about three times more likely to have lung cancer, identified either through hospitalization records or mortality records. Of the people who developed, or died of, lung cancer, those with six or more adverse events in childhood were roughly 13 years younger at presentation than those with none. People who had experienced more adverse events in childhood showed more smoking behaviors," Brown was quoted as saying.

The central message of this study is that our children can be faced with a terrible burden of stressors. These stressors are associated with harmful behaviors, such as smoking, which may lead the development of diseases like lung cancer and perhaps death at a younger age. Reducing the burden of adverse childhood experiences should therefore be considered in health and social programs as a means of primary prevention of lung cancer and other smoking-related diseases. (SOURCE: BMC Public Health, January 18, 2010)

What these studies show us is that having trauma early in our lives may set us up for thinking patterns and behavior patterns that may be conducive to disease. This does not mean that everyone who had early childhood trauma will have a disease later in life, but, it does mean that people who do have early trauma have a higher incidence of having a disease.

Why? Well, again, how we react to the stress and the traumas of our lives will make all the difference to our health.

Let's continue on and begin to look at what the medical community knows about our thoughts and how they affect our health. There is actually an area of study that is called:

Psychoneuroimmunolgy

How one reacts to stress appears to be a major factor in the development of cancer. Most cancer patients have experienced a highly stressful event, usually about two-years prior to the onset of detectable disease. This traumatic event is often beyond the patient's control, such as the loss of a loved one, loss of a business, job, home, or some other major disaster. The typical cancer victim has lost the ability to cope with these extreme events, because his/her coping mechanism lies in his/her ability to control the environment. When this control is lost, the patient has no other way to cope.

Major stress, as we have seen, causes suppression of the immune system, and does so more overwhelmingly in the cancer-susceptible individual than in others. Thus personal tragedies and excessive levels of stress appear to combine with the underlying personality described above to bring on the immune deficiency which allows cancer to thrive. As quoted in the Cancer Personality[23] research.

These observations have given rise to the term psychoneuroimmunology.

Let's define this term:

Psychoneuroimmunology (PNI)[24] is the study of the interaction between psychological processes and the nervous and immune systems of the human body.

PNI is a branch of medicine that deals with the influence of emotional states (as stress) and nervous system activities on immune function especially in relation to the onset and progression of disease.

To understand the term PNI, we can start by breaking it into and defining the component parts:

Psyche - the mind component or study of psychology, the cognitive and emotional processes involving mood states.

Neuro - the neurologic connections e.g. neurotransmitters and neuroendocrine secretions, or study of neurology components is impacted, or the study of immunology.

Immunology - how the immune system e.g. the cellular and humoral.

Research is adding importance to this field of study[24]:

The current research in the field of PNI is demonstrating the inter-connections of the mind, the body and the spirit. One is no longer able to focus on the mind as an abstract phenomenon that is separate from the processes of the body and the emotions. The health or well-being of the body can no longer ignore the impact of the mind, the emotions or the spirit on the process.

In simple terms this is the study of how our thoughts, feelings, emotions and beliefs can affect the functioning of our immune systems and our body and ultimately our health.

The medical community knows that this is true and they have an entire section of study devoted to researching the connection between what we think, feel and believe and do, with how our bodies work.

This study of medicine coincides with our understanding of God's word that tells us that how we think and behave will determine the health of our bodies and our minds.

Here is a quote from Hippocrates: *"It is more important to know what sort of person has a disease than to know what sort of disease a person has."*

What Hippocrates is saying is that it is very important to know what a person is thinking and feeling and doing, because that may be the very key to the person's healing.

In short, PNI is the study of the connection between our body and our mind. This is where the medical community studies how our thoughts, beliefs, feelings and attitudes can affect the health of our bodies.

This is a medical dictionary definition of this scientific study:

Medical Dictionary: psy·cho·neu·ro·im·mu·nol·o·gy definition: Pronunciation: /j/ Function: n-pl-gies; a field of medicine that deals with the influence of emotional states (as stress) and nervous system activity on immune function especially in relation to their effect on the onset and progression of disease.

There is also another medical diagnosis that is the psychological community's diagnosis of *somatization disorder.* This disorder also points to thoughts becoming symptoms in our bodies.

So·mat·i·cize Psychiatry - to convert (anxiety) into physical symptoms. Somatoform disorders are characterized by physical disorders from stress and anxiety.

"Somatoform disorders are characterized by a concern with the body. Stress and trauma lead to anxiety, but instead of developing one of the anxiety disorders or depression, some people somaticize: They experience the anxiety as fatigue, loss of appetite, body aches, headaches, gastrointestinal problems, and so on. Somatization is actually the most common manifestation of anxiety, especially in non-western countries."

"In China, somatization disorder is a relatively common problem, and is labelled neurasthenia. Neurasthenia combines somatization with feelings of anxiety, depression, irritability, and distraction. In Korea, there is a version called hwa-byung ("anger illness"). It is most commonly

71

found in less educated, middle aged women who are trapped in bad marriages[25]."

This is the medical community's evaluation of how we are somaticizing our anxieties and stresses into physical illnesses and symptoms. With the study of psychoneuroimmunology and with the somatoform disorder, the medical community gains perspective on the mind and body connection.

God Speaks To Us About Our Health

These studies just open our eyes to the definite connection that exists between our mind and our body. As children of God, we also know that we have another dimension to our creation and that is our spirit. I wanted to interject this section here, but will be talking more on God and His thoughts later in this book.

Our spirit man is how we communicate with God. We have a mind, a spirit and we live in a human body. While we are on this planet, we need our body to house our spirit and soul.

We also know that what we allow to hang out in our mind and in our spirit is what we can see reflected in our body by health or disease. In other words, our bodies will show what we think about in our minds.

Let's look at a scripture that can prove this:

3 John 2 *Beloved, I wish above all things that thou mayest prosper and be in health, even as thy soul prospereth.*

What does this scripture mean? To the degree of our soul health is our physical health.

The scripture lets us know that as your soul prospers—and your soul is where you think, make decisions, have your will and your memories—as your soul prospers, or aligns with God and His word, your body will be in health or keep well.

God is telling us that what you think and believe and do will determine how healthy your body is.

Proverbs 23:7 *For as he thinketh in his heart, so is he.*

What you think can determine who you are, and it can determine how healthy your body is.

God has told us so many times that our health depends on what we think and how we behave.

I am sharing these studies and articles with you because I want to make sure that you know that God told us that what you think and how you behave is what will determine the health of your body. I also want you to see that man and science is beginning to show that this is true also.

God's word is truth. The Bible tells us that the truth can set you free. However, the truth can only set you free when you are exposed to the truth, when you listen to the truth and when you believe the truth and when you decide to live by the truth.

John 8:32 *And ye shall know the truth, and the truth shall make you free.*

The word "know" means the following: To know, understand, perceive, and have knowledge of.

The truth means this—that which is true in things appertaining to God and the duties of man, moral and religious truth.

The words "make you free" means this—to set at liberty from the dominion of sin. Just reading the word will not necessarily set you free. It means knowing and understanding the word, it is walking in the word. It is applying the truth of the word to your life. What sets us free is truly living by the word of God.

James 1:22 *But be ye doers of the word, and not hearers only, deceiving your own selves.*

We have to hear the word and do the word in our daily lives. See, we can go to church every Sunday, we can go to church Wednesday night, we can talk Christian-eze, we can have a bumper sticker and a Jesus pin, we can even cast out devils, but, we can be missing the true impact of the gospel which is teaching us how to think and behave and how to have relationships with other people with ourselves and with God.

Matthew 7:21-23 *Not everyone that saith unto me, Lord, Lord, shall enter into the kingdom of heaven; but he that doeth the will of my Father which is in heaven. ²²Many will say to me in that day, Lord, Lord, have we not prophesied in thy name? and in thy name have cast out devils? and in thy name done many wonderful works? ²³And then will I profess unto them, I never knew you: depart from me, ye that work iniquity.*

God wants us to be hearers and doers of the word. He wants us to study His word and His ways so that we have wisdom and knowledge. He wants us to apply His word to our everyday lives and in everything that we think and do. He wants us to have healthy lives and since He created us, He knows what it will take to be healthy.

We have problems because of our own lack of knowledge. We don't really know how to think and behave properly.

> **Hosea 4:6** *My people are destroyed for lack of knowledge: because thou hast rejected knowledge, I will also reject thee, that thou shalt be no priest to me: seeing thou hast forgotten the law of thy God, I will also forget thy children.*

If we have a lack of knowledge, this lack of knowledge falls on us and our children. Our ancestor's lack of knowledge of God and His word has affected us.

> **Isaiah 5:13** *Therefore my people are gone into captivity, because they have no knowledge.*

We are being held captive because we have no knowledge. The bottom line is that we don't know how to think and behave like Jesus did when He was on this planet. We don't know how to think and behave in the ways that God tells us about in the Bible.

So, we know that God tells us all about how our thoughts and behaviors affect our health and our very life. In reality, God talks about psychoneuroimmunology in His word!

God's Study of Psychoneuroimmunology

Let's look at some scriptures that tell us all about the connection between our thoughts and behaviors and our health.

Did you know that a disease can't come into your life without a cause?

Proverbs 26:2 *As a bird by wondering and a swallow by flying, so the curse causeless shall not come.*

God tells us that there is a mind, spirit and body connection.

Proverbs 23:7 *As a man thinketh in his heart, so is he.*

When we have no hope, we can get sick.

Proverbs 13:12 *Hope deferred makes the heart sick.*

Being happy is like taking medicine.

Proverbs 17:22 *A merry heart doeth good like a medicine.*

Here is a connection between your spirit and the health of your body.

Proverbs 17:22 *A broken spirit drieth up the bones.*

Here is a connection between your thoughts and your bones where your immune system is created.

Proverbs 14:30 *A sound heart is the life of the flesh: but envy the rottenness of the bones.*

When we trust the Lord, we can be happy.

Proverbs 16:20 *He that handleth a matter wisely shall find good: and whoso trusteth in the LORD, happy is he.*

Here is a connection between your health and what you say.

Proverbs 18:21 *Death and life are in the power of the tongue.*

These are just a few of the scriptures in the Bible that connect our thoughts to the health of our bodies. God knows about psychoneuroimmunology! He told us about the connection between our spirit, soul and body in the Bible.

Your Health and Thoughts

We are talking about cancer in this book, but the truth is that no matter what your disease process is, the same truths that we will talk about that relate to God in terms of cancer can apply to other diseases.

Let's move along with some more articles and studies that the medical community has written and published that show us direct connections between how we think and behave and diseases that have a right to our bodies:

Mind Over Cancer by author Michelle Hancock[26]

Not a day goes by that the word "cancer" doesn't scare thousands of Canadians. Like a dreaded scourge, it hovers over us, presumably just waiting to claim its next victim. But according to scientists in the growing field of mind/body medicine, the disease is not as much an external force as you might believe. Fear and anxiety–our thoughts and feelings–can impact our health just as much as a long list of cancer risk factors.

"Psychoneuroimmunology"' is the scientific term to describe the study of the mind/body connection. Carl Simonton, MD, is an oncologist who pioneered research in this discipline as early as the 1970s. His book, Getting Well Again (Bantam, 1978), shows how "an individual's reaction to stress and other emotional factors can contribute to the onset and progress of cancer [while] positive expectations, self-awareness and self-care can contribute to survival."

Isn't it interesting that this tells us that fear can hurt our immune systems to the point of allowing a disease process to begin in our bodies. Fear and stress can also allow the disease to progress once you have been diagnosed with the disease.

One thing that I know is that fear and stress is always listed as the number one issue when we consider spiritual roots to disease as noted in "A More Excellent Way."

Fear comes into our lives when we have doubt and unbelief in God.

The interesting thing is that we are so fearfully and wonderfully made by God—our Creator—that He knows how we have to think and behave so that our bodies will work optimally and support us in health and not disease.

Hebrews 11:6 *But without faith it is impossible to please Him: for he that cometh to God must believe that He is, and that He is a rewarder of them that diligently seek Him.*

By teaching us all about these issues, God has opened up an entire new dimension of life to us. He is giving us important information about how He created us. He created us to be in health or to be healthy—when we have faith.

What is fear? It is the opposite of faith. When you have faith, fear cannot be executed in your mind. The opposite is true, as well. If you are entertaining fear, faith cannot be executed.

Only one thing, fear or faith can be what you believe at any moment in time. And, if you are in fear you secrete chemicals that create an environment in your body that is conducive to symptoms and disease.

Here is the thing to remember, God knows that if you entertain an evil spirit of fear you are not in faith.

Here is a scripture that tells us about this:

2 Timothy 1:7 *For God hath not given us the spirit of fear; but of power, and of love, and of a sound mind.*

God did not give us a spirit of fear. This spirit of fear is an evil spirit of fear. God gives us love, power and a sound mind. Remember, a spirit of fear is not your friend.

He did not give us the fear that opens up the doors to Satan and his kingdom. When we agree and listen to Satan and his kingdom, he can influence us to think and behave in ways that create a chemical environment in our bodies where disease can flourish.

Here is another study that equates personality and cancer. As you read this article and I present the personality issues that Dr. Brodie saw, remember that I am going to discuss these issues in relation to God later in this book.

Causes of Cancer: The Cancer Personality by W. Douglas Brodie, MD[27].

In dealing with many thousands of cancer patients over the past 28 years, it has been my observation that there are certain personality traits present in the cancer-susceptible individual.

These traits are as follows:

1. Being highly conscientious, caring, dutiful, responsible, hard-working, and usually of above average intelligence. (My comment: performance and perfection)
2. Exhibits a strong tendency toward carrying other people's burdens and toward taking on extra obligations, and often "worrying for others." (My comment: False burden bearing)

3. Having a deep-seated need to make others happy. Being a "people pleaser" with a great need for approval. (My comment: Fabrication, control, manipulation, Jezebel characteristics)

4. Often lacking closeness with one or both parents, which sometimes, later in life, results in lack of closeness with spouse or others who would normally be close. (my comment: Fear of intimacy and lack of relationship skills, a self focus)

5. Harbors long-suppressed toxic emotions, such as anger, resentment and/or hostility. The cancer-susceptible individual typically internalizes such emotions and has great difficulty expressing them. (My comment: Spirit of bitterness, holding a record of wrongs, denial, lack of relationship skills)

6. Reacts adversely to stress, and often becomes unable to cope adequately with such stress. Usually experiences an especially damaging event about 2 years before the onset of detectable cancer. The patient is not able to cope with this traumatic event or series of events, which comes as a "last straw" on top of years of suppressed reactions to stress. (My comment: Bitterness, broken heart, broken spirit, doubt and unbelief in God)

7. Has an inability to resolve deep-seated emotional problems and conflicts, usually beginning in childhood, often even being unaware of their presence. (My comment: Denial and lack of Godly skills)

Typical of the cancer-susceptible personality, as noted above, is the long-standing tendency to suppress "toxic emotions," particularly anger. Usually beginning in childhood, this individual has held in their hostility and other unacceptable emotions. More often than not, this feature of the affected personality has its origins in feelings of rejection by one or both parents. Whether these feelings of rejection are justified or not, the individual perceives this rejection as real, and this results in a lack of closeness with the "rejecting" parent, followed later in life by a lack of closeness with spouses and others with whom close relationships would normally develop. Those at the higher risk for cancer tend to develop feelings of loneliness as a result of their having been deprived of affection and acceptance earlier in life, even if this is only their perception. They have a tremendous need for approval and acceptance, and develop a very high sensitivity to the needs of others while suppressing their own emotional needs.

They become the "caretakers" of the world, showing great compassion and caring for others, and will go out of their way to look after others. They are very reluctant to accept help from others, fearing that it may jeopardize their role as the caretaker. Throughout their childhood they have been typically taught "not to be selfish", and they take this to heart as a major lifetime objective. All of this is highly commendable in our culture, but must be somehow modified in the case of the cancer patient. A distinction needs to be made here between the "care-giving" and the "care-taking" personality. There is nothing wrong with care-giving, of course, but the problem arises when the susceptible individual derives their entire worth, value and identity from their role as "caretaker." If this very important shift cannot be made, the patient is stuck in this role, and the susceptibility to cancer greatly increases.

As already stated, a consistent feature of those who are susceptible to cancer appears to be that they "suffer in silence", and bear their burdens without complaint. These burdens of their own as well as the burdens of others weigh heavily upon these people through a lifetime of emotional suppression. The carefree extrovert, on the other hand, seems to be far less vulnerable to cancer than the caring introvert described above.

How one reacts to stress appears to be a major factor in the larger number of contributing causes of cancer. Most cancer patients have experienced a highly stressful event, usually about 2 years prior to the onset of detectable disease. This traumatic event is often beyond the patient's control, such as the loss of a loved one, loss of a business, job, home, or some other major disaster. The typical cancer personality has lost the ability to cope with these extreme events, because his/her coping mechanism lies in his/her ability to control the environment. When this control is lost, the patient has no other way to cope.

Major stress causes suppression of the immune system, and does so more overwhelmingly in the cancer-susceptible individual than in others. Thus personal tragedies and excessive levels of stress appear to combine with the underlying personality described above to bring on the immune deficiency which allows cancer to thrive.

Here is some more information that goes along with what we just read. Dr. Jürgen Buche lucidly observes[28]:

> (Cancer) patients do not want to die or suffer but they have no compelling purpose for LIVING. They submit passively to regimes and procedures to please their families or their physician but they spiral uncomplainingly downward. The litmus question to a cancer or AIDS patient "What real reason do you have for living?" is often unanswerable. The will to live must come from the patient and no amount of anguish, encouragement or threats from any family or friends will help if this will to live is not present. Often, such a situation is intimately linked to a lack of love."

These statements that we see in what Dr. Buche has written, follow scripture, as well. Without a vision for our future, one can lose the will to live. Here is a scripture that tells us the same thing.

Proverbs 29:18 *Where there is no vision, the people perish.*

When we don't have a vision for our future, we can let a spirit of hopelessness and a spirit of death have access to our lives. We can become hopeless and think that we have no purpose in our lives. We may think that we have nothing to look forward to or that we have no goals. We can lose excitement for our lives. We may not think that we have a purpose for our lives.

This scripture is telling us that when we have no goals or visions for our future, people perish or die. We have to be very careful about listening to thoughts about hopelessness. We have to actively pursue goals, visions or dreams for our future that line up with God and His word.

Psalm 37:4 *Delight thyself also in the LORD: and he shall give thee the desires of thine heart.*

When we are hearers and doers of God's word, He will give us Godly desires in our hearts. Out of our relationship with our Father in heaven, our hearts will be filled with Godly desires.

God would never leave us without a Godly vision for our future. He has good plans for us!

Jeremiah 29:11 *For I know the thoughts that I think toward you, saith the LORD, thoughts of peace, and not of evil, to give you an expected end.*

Another important issue to understand is that God created us for love and relationship with Him and with others and with ourselves. When we are lacking that love, we can look for love in all the wrong places. When we don't find the love in the wrong places, we can lose our will to live. We can lose our hopes and dreams and goals for the future.

This is Satan's plan for our lives. This can let a spirit of hopelessness, infirmity and death into our lives.

Here is some more information that I think is important to know about thoughts and hopelessness:

The Power of Belief II[29] by Mike Beebe (reproduced by Healing Cancer Naturally with permission of the author)

Deepak Chopra tells a story about a medical doctor who had not had a check up for 25 years. (Physician! Heal thyself!) When he was compelled to get a physical due to life insurance requirements, a large dark spot was found on his lung. It was diagnosed as inoperable cancer. The doc died a couple of months later. Some days after the funeral, Chopra was sorting through the physician's effects and came across a chest x-ray that was 25 years old. Out of curiosity, he put it up to the light and, lo and behold, there was that same dark spot on the lung! The deceased doctor had lived a vigorous life all those years and was, in effect, killed by the diagnosis and not the disease.

This story confirms what the Bible says:

Proverbs 23:7 *For as he thinketh in his heart, so is he.*

This man lost hope. He thought he was sick and dying, and that is just what he did. Remember: think sick, be sick. What we think about and agree with can become truth for us. That is why God tells us to watch all of our thoughts and hold them captive. He tells us to compare all of our thoughts with His words in the Bible. If what we are thinking about does not line up with God's word, we are told to cast down those thoughts. God tells us this because what we think about is what we believe and what can become true for us.

2 Corinthians 10:5 *Casting down imaginations, and every high thing that exalteth itself against the knowledge of God, and bringing into captivity every thought to the obedience of Christ.*

We have to watch all of our thoughts, and if they don't agree with God and His word, we cast them down and get rid of them. We make a choice to exchange them with thoughts and beliefs that come from the word of God.

We can see that some researchers and doctors in the medical community have defined specific character/behavior traits that people with cancer seem to have. However, these researchers don't seem to understand God and His word and how these traits relate to God and His kingdom. They don't seem to know how to work these issues out with God.

Later in this book I am going to reframe these traits considering God and His word and I am also going to explain Godly ways to handle these issues.

The Medical Community and God

This last article we reviewed is so interesting and true. When we feel deprived, when we feel empty or depressed, or incomplete, or hopeless or unloved or we are just feeling badly, we can begin to have addictions. We can be addicted to gambling or another person. We can be addicted to bad relationships, we can be addicted to sex, or we can be addicted to attention, or we can be addicted to being sick, or we can be addicted to doctors, or prescription drugs, or recreational and illegal drugs. We can be addicted to alcohol or we can be addicted to spending money or shopping sprees or eating or we can be addicted to not eating. The truth is that we can be addicted to almost anything.

When we don't feel whole, we try to fill ourselves up with anything that can make us feel better – even if it is just for a moment. We are all the while not looking for the true God that can fill us with His truth and with His love. We can be unaware that in our relationship with God, is where we can find wholeness.

The medical community knows what the personality problems are that can lead to disease, but they don't know the one true God who sent His word to heal us and deliver us from our own destructions.

The only thing that the medical community can do when a diagnosis of cancer is made is to offer surgery and medication, chemotherapy and radiation. These kinds of cancer treatments target the tumor by killing the cancer cells or by removing the tumor. However, radiation, chemotherapy and surgery are not preventive strategies. They target the tumor itself. They may not prevent the tumor from recurring or growing back. The other important issue is that they may not kill the cancer cells that are responsible for the tumors. These treatments do nothing to deal with the roots that allowed the cancer to begin in the first place.

Sometimes support groups or counseling are offered so that the person can try to better handle the issues in their lives caused by the disease process. Sometimes people go to alternative doctors and they can get lots of supplements, vitamins, vitamin IV's and alternative medicines and practices like aromatherapy or Homeopathy. You might even be offered chiropractic manipulation, acupuncture or psychiatry.

But, if your disease process began because of the way that you think and behave, how can you really expect to be cured of cancer if you don't change the way that you think and behave? The most that you can hope for is to manage the disease and hope to get healed by something that the doctors do.

If the environment in your body is created by your thoughts and your behaviors and you continue to think and behave in the same ways that created the environment in your body that was conducive to cancer, your immune system will continue to be weakened or dysfunctional.

Following is some more information about medical doctors and cancer.

The Cancer Personality: Its Importance in Healing by W. Douglas Brodie, MD[30].

In my experience, one of the most difficult and most important hurdles to overcome in cancer patients is how to make major changes in their life-styles. Not only is it necessary to make changes in the physical aspects of their lives such as eating habits, but major changes need to be made in the way they react to stress. The way they react to stress is due largely to the way they think about life. There can be no lasting changes of behavior without first having a change in thinking and in belief systems. It is often extremely difficult for these patients to make substantial changes in these ingrained patterns of thought. Many find it too difficult or too disagreeable to make such alterations in their settled way of thinking and reacting. Many likewise find it too unpleasant to make changes in the physical aspects of their life-style, even in the face of life-threatening illness.

In my office patients are counseled to address their problems and to make the appropriate adjustments to the best of their ability. A psychologist with extensive experience in dealing with these unique problems is readily available to our patients."

This doctor's opinion is that in order for the cancer patient to get well, the cancer patients have to change their lives and their thinking and behavior patterns. They have to have changes in their belief systems. Dr. Brodie's observation is that they have to make major changes in their lives.

Dr. Lothar Hirneise[31] noticed "something else" in every case that he saw where people were healed of cancer.

But I noticed something else. I call it SYSTEM CHANGE. We all live in Systems, in our marriage, in our house, in our job, etc. Many, many, many of these cancer patients made system jumps. They kicked their husband in the butt and threw him out. They quit their job, they moved, they not only moved their bed, they moved out of their apartment, they went to other countries. Does it mean that you have to do all of these things? I don't know. Quite honestly, I don't know. But I can tell you from my experience, it's just remarkable to what extent people changed their life before they were in a position to get well.

Dr. Bodo Kohler wrote in his book that he was almost sure that he could heal any cancer patient. How? "I take him by the hand and fly him to an oasis in Africa. Let's see whether the tumor can survive this. Now what happens in an oasis? The sun?—sure, the sun can help. But something else is more important. When you have cancer and you fly to an oasis in Africa you have more or less left all the systems in which you live here. And this makes it difficult for a tumor to survive in your body."

This is what I think is the most revealing information. This doctor saw that people got well when they changed the way that they interacted in their lives. They changed the way that they interacted with their family and they changed the way that they thought. The truth is that they changed just about everything.

When I first got really sick in 1987, I had a doctor whom I asked this question, "Have you ever seen anyone that got better from what I have?" He said, "Yes. I saw one person get well. But this person changed their whole life, everything, they moved far away and they left their old life and they changed everything and they got well."

At the time all of those years ago when I heard this, I was confused. I did not know what this meant. I did not even have the first clue about what I had to change in order to get well.

Today, I do know a little about what this means. It means that we have to be sanctified, we have to change and be transformed by God and His word. We have to leave our old lives behind and move into our new lives—with God. We have to leave our old thoughts, beliefs and behaviors behind and replace them with new ones that line up with God. We have to leave our past behind and move into our future as new men and women with God.

The end result will be that we have new thoughts, beliefs and behaviors that line up with God and His word.

Here are some scriptures that we can relate to these changes.

2 Corinthians 5:17 *Therefore if any man be in Christ, he is a new creature: old things are passed away; behold, all things are become new.*

Ephesians 4:24 *And that ye put on the new man, which after God is created in righteousness and true holiness.*

Colossians 3:10 *And have put on the new man, which is renewed in knowledge after the image of him that created him:*

In my own life, just about everything changed. I got saved and then God worked with me to change. The changes took a long time and it was a process – not an overnight event.

Here is another scripture that teaches us about transformation and change.

Romans 12:2 *And be not conformed to this world: but be ye transformed by the renewing of your mind, that ye may prove what is that good, and acceptable, and perfect, will of God.*

When we enter into a real and intimate relationship with God, we are signing up for change. We are going to be changed by the word.

Our relationship with God is all about behavior modification. When we are in right relationship with God and within our self, as He designed us to be, we can experience healthy behavior modification], We have to renew our minds to think as God thinks so that we can walk in His word and in His ways. When our thoughts change, our feelings, beliefs and actions will change.

What the scripture tells us is that we have to change our old ways to new ways. We have to let go of the past and walk into our present and future with God.

Here is another article that has some pertinent information. I quote comments from Andreas Moritz in his article:

"Cancer is Not a Disease – It's a Survival Mechanism" that present challenging thinking about cancer and its healing.

Cancer has always been an extremely rare illness, except in industrialized nations during the past 40-50 years. Human genes have not significantly changed for thousands of years. Why would they change so drastically now, and suddenly decide to kill scores of people? The answer to this question is amazingly simple: Damaged or faulty genes do not kill anyone. Cancer does not kill a person afflicted with it! What kills a cancer patient is not the tumor, but the numerous reasons behind cell mutation and tumor growth. These root causes should be the focus of every cancer treatment, yet most oncologists typically ignore them. Constant conflicts, guilt and shame, for example, can easily paralyze the body's most basic functions, and lead to the growth of a cancerous tumor.

After having seen thousands of cancer patients over a period of three decades, I began to recognize a certain pattern of thinking, believing and feeling that was common to most of them. To be more specific, I have yet to meet a cancer patient who does not feel burdened by some poor self-image, unresolved conflict and worries, or past emotional trauma that still lingers in his/her subconscious. Cancer, the physical disease, cannot occur unless there is a strong undercurrent of emotional uneasiness and deep-seated frustration.

Cancer patients typically suffer from lack of self-respect or worthiness, and often have what I call an "unfinished business" in their life. Cancer can actually be a way of revealing the source of such inner conflict. Furthermore, cancer can help them come to terms with such a conflict, and even heal it altogether. The way to take out weeds is to pull them out along with their roots. This is how we must treat cancer; otherwise, it may recur eventually.

The following statement is very important in the consideration of cancer: "Cancer does not cause a person to be sick; it is the sickness of the person that causes the cancer[32]. To treat cancer successfully requires the patient to become whole again on all levels of his body, mind and spirit. Once the cancer causes have been properly identified, it will become apparent what needs to be done to achieve complete recovery.

We all know that if the foundation of a house is strong the house can easily withstand external challenges such as a violent storm. As we will see, cancer is merely an indication that there is something missing in our body and in life as a whole. Cancer shows that life as a whole (physical, mental and spiritual) stands on shaky grounds and is quite fragile, to say the least. It would be foolish for a gardener to water the withering leaves of a tree when he knows so well that the real problem is not where it appears to be, namely, on the symptomatic level (of withered leaves). By watering the roots of the plant, he naturally attends to the causative level, and consequently, the plant regenerates itself swiftly and automatically.

This article offers the rather bizarre theory that the reason that cancer can kill is not the cancer itself. The problem and question to ask can be said to be this—what is it about the person's body that is allowing the cancer to grow and proliferate? The author, who is not a medical doctor but a practitioner of Ayurveda, iridology, shiatsu, a writer, and an artist who has studied holistic healing, gives his answer to this when he mentions that constant conflicts, guilt and shame can be responsible for paralyzing or stopping our bodies from working properly.

We see this author relating lack of self-respect and feeling unworthy as a characteristic of the person's personality that can lead to disease. This is consistent with the cancer personality profiles that we see emerging. If we treat symptoms and not the real reason or root of the symptoms, we are not treating the origin of the disease. We are just chasing symptoms. We are just trying to manage symptoms. We are not getting to the root of the problem. All of these articles and studies show us that we all have a lot to learn about how to get to the roots of our problems.

Cancer is the fruit of some root. In order to get well, we have to recognize what the root to the disease is and deal with it with God. We have to change! Be transformed! We have to be willing to change what is making us sick. Getting healed is all about change and transformation. We have to become whole in body, mind and spirit.

How do we begin to do this? God tells us how in this next scripture.

Psalm 139:23-4 *Search me, O God, and know my heart; test me and know my anxious thoughts. See if there is any offensive way in me, and lead me in the way everlasting.*

In this Psalm, David was talking to God and asking Him to show him what is really going on in his heart and to lead him in God's ways which are eternal and everlasting. This is exactly what I want to do in this book. I want to expose the thoughts and behaviors that we have that are not lining up with God and His word.

We need to learn about spiritual roots that lead to disease.

Spiritual Roots and Cancer

These articles and medical studies that we have been reviewing, can show us that the way that a person thinks and behaves can lead to a propensity to allowing a disease into our lives.

One of the comments we read by Andreas Moritz was, *"Cancer does not cause a person to be sick; it is the sickness of the person that causes the cancer."* Moritz went on to say, *"To treat cancer successfully requires the patient to become whole again on all levels of his body, mind and spirit."*

We can extrapolate about this and say that there are roots or reasons why people get cancer and these roots or reasons can start in the person's soul or spirit. The roots or reasons that the person's body was susceptible to cancer in the first place can be caused by the way that the person thinks, believes and behaves. When we look at people who have a disease process in their bodies, we can say that they have spiritual roots to the disease process. Spiritual roots to a disease can be defined as roots to our physical diseases that come from our thinking and behaviors and our spiritual life.

Our spiritual life is our relationship with God and His word, our relationship with ourselves and our relationship with other people. Our spiritual roots are the problems that we have in our thoughts and our behaviors, our beliefs and our relationships that don't line up with God and His word. If we are sick and dying, we can look for spiritual problems in our lives that might be contributing to our disease.

Let's look again at the Mortiz quote about treating cancer, *"To treat cancer successfully requires the patient to become whole again on all levels of his body, mind and spirit."*

We can extrapolate from this comment and say that to treat a disease successfully, it requires the patient to become whole again on all levels of his creation. We must become whole in our mind and in our spirit and that can translate to health in our body.

When we are sick, and we have symptoms in our bodies or in our minds, we often look to the medical community and the doctor to help us and to stop our sickness and our symptoms.

Let me give you an example of why looking at the physical symptoms and trying to get cured with physical remedies won't help to find the real reason or the root to why you got sick in the first place.

This is a true story that I would like to use to make a point. In 2010, I walked into my mother's house and found myself ankle deep in water in the kitchen. I looked around and saw nothing obvious that would cause the flood. I could not find the root of the flood. I did see water all over the place, so I knew that the water had to be coming from some place. I knew that the water was the fruit of some root, so I figured that it might be the obvious and

I reached under the sink and I closed the water valves that were coming into the sink. I figured that this action would stop the water from continuing to flood the kitchen. My next reaction was to clean the water up. I went into the garage and I got paper towels and old newspapers and I began to clean up the mess. The more that I cleaned up the water the more water was coming onto the floor. I just kept wiping up the floor. Then I began to realize that there was another root to the water and I had better find the root or the real reason for the flood. I realized that I had to locate the problem and stop it, or else the kitchen would continue to flood.

Even though I was trying to care of the symptom—the flood—I needed to know what the root to the flood was so that I could stop it from continuing. So, I went outside and I closed the water valve that allowed water into the whole house. Now the flooding stopped.

There is more to this story. I called a friend and he helped me to clean the water up. We called a plumber and continued to clean the water. But something told me to look in the room that has its wall next to the kitchen—it was a bedroom—and I walked in there to ankle deep water. I realized that the problem was much more widespread than I had realized and that we had a real problem.

Eventually we found that there was a pipe in the wall that broke, and it had caused the house to flood. The root to the problem was the broken pipe. I tried to fix the problem at first by cleaning up the water. But because I did not find the root to the problem—the pipe—the water kept flooding.

I tried to clean up the water and I was doing okay, but the water slowly kept coming onto the floor. I was putting a band-aid on the problem. In order to completely stop the problem I needed to find the root of the problem and fix the root.

This is a metaphor for our lives. If we have symptoms in our bodies or we have a sickness or a disease and we try to fix the disease by using drugs and medicines and other medical modalities, we are not fixing the root problem or the reason why we got the disease or symptom in the first place.

We are just managing symptoms. We are not getting to the real reason why our body manifested these symptoms in the first place. We are not getting to the root of the problem and trying to fix the root.

The spiritual root to our problems can come from not having healthy relationships with God or ourselves or with other people.

Our thinking and our behaviors and our ability to have healthy relationships can be at the root to our diseases. Some examples of spiritual roots to disease can be fear, anxiety, stress, bitterness, un-forgiveness, resentment, holding grudges, gossip, murder, rejection, envy, jealousy, rebellion, fabricating our personality, striving, problems with self esteem and not being able to identify and feel our feelings properly. We can be lying to ourselves and to God and not even know that any of these things could be causing our problems.

There are many more spiritual roots to our diseases, these are just examples, but these give you an idea of where to start looking for roots to diseases in your life.

When we look at spiritual roots we can learn things about ourselves that can help us to work with God about our sin issues. When we work with God we have an opportunity to change those patterns of thinking and behaving that can lead to an open door to Satan and his kingdom and a disease process.

We have stated earlier that if we have a disease process in our bodies there can be spiritual roots to the disease. In other words, we can have ways of thinking and believing and we can have attitudes and behaviors that do not line up with God and His word. This thinking that does not line up with God and His word can be a root or a reason why we have sickness and disease in our bodies and our minds.

If you trust the doctors for your healing, and you have spiritual roots to your disease, you may have a problem. You may be managing symptoms instead of finding the root to your problems.

God tells us about trusting in something other than Him and His word.

Psalm 20:7 says, *Some trust in chariots, and some in horses: but we will remember the name of the LORD our God.*

We can extrapolate and say "some trust in doctors, some trust in chiropractors, some trust in acupuncture, some trust in vitamins, some trust in medicines, but we—the children of the most high God—will trust in the name of the LORD our God and in His creative design for our bodies and environment."

If we are trying to kill the cancer, but our body has an environment that is conducive to disease and cancer because of our thoughts, beliefs and attitudes, then we are trying to bypass the curse of the disease without addressing the real root to the disease. In other words, we want to get rid of the disease without dealing with the original root, or the reason why we got the disease in the first place.

Disease is a Curse

How do we know this?

In Deuteronomy 28 and Leviticus 26, God reveals blessings and cursings to us. Scripture tells us that if we obey God and walk in His word and in His ways, we will be blessed and if we don't, curses can come into our lives. If we study these scriptures, we can see that the listings of curses are diseases and situations.

In Deuteronomy 7:12-15 God tells us that if we listen to His word and we line up with His word and His ways, that he will bless us, even by taking away the diseases that our disobedience had caused.

The root to our problems is that we are not being hearers and doers of God's word.

James 1:22 *But be ye doers of the word, and not hearers only, deceiving your own selves.*

The root is that we don't know how to think and behave according to God and His word so that we can have a healthy mind and body. The root is that we don't know how to have relationships with God, with other people and with ourselves. This is the biggest problem that people can have—we don't know how to have healthy, Godly relationships.

Simply put, we do not know how to think and behave in the ways that our Creator has laid out for us in the Bible. Remember, if our thoughts and behaviors line up with Satan and his kingdom, we can have an environment in our body that supports cancer and/or any disease process.

I want to make one point clear; I am not saying that we should not pursue medical treatments; I am saying that the most important thing that we should pursue is our healthy relationship with God and His ways. The most important thing that we should pursue is God and His word—that is found in the Bible. What is our goal? We want to have a healthy mind, body and spirit.

Psalm 119:11 *Thy word have I hid in mine heart, that I might not sin against thee.*

If we don't know the word of God and we don't have it hidden in our hearts, we can be allowing toxic and deadly thoughts and emotions to hang around in our minds. This can create an environment in our bodies that is going to allow sickness and disease flourish. In this study about cancer, I am going to discuss those patterns of thinking and behaving that seem to be involved in creating the environment in the body that allows cancer to grow.

Character Traits

The next thing that I would like to do is to begin to discuss the specific roots or the character traits that we can see in someone who has cancer. In the next section, we will look at some of the character traits that someone has before the diagnosis of cancer and then we will discuss what happens after the diagnosis.

There are a lot of things that can happen after the doctor gives us a medical diagnosis, and we will discuss those issues. But, first let's look at how Satan and his kingdom have influenced people to think and behave and how that can lead to disease in the first place.

When I presented the articles and studies at the beginning of this book, we saw that the medical community has identified some definite character traits that can be seen in someone who has developed cancer.

We could say briefly what the medical community has said that the person who has a Type C personality "is a feeling denier, avoider, suppressor, or repressor. They may be a stoic, they may fabricate their personality and they can tend to be a false burden bearer. He or she can have a calm, outwardly rational, and unemotional demeanor, but also a tendency to conform to the wishes of others, a lack of assertiveness, and an inclination toward feelings of helplessness or hopelessness."

They can be angry. They can be depressed. They can be hopeless and they may not have a vision for their future.

I just want to mention that the medical community says that the root to depression is unexpressed feelings of anger. Through many years of study, I have found that depression can be covering up all kinds of feelings—not just anger. People can have feelings of fear, sadness, disappointment, loneliness, embarrassment, anger, resentment, envy and jealousy or any kind of thoughts and feelings that are denied and not dealt with.

From working with people who have cancer I have seen that these personality traits are accurate to a great degree.

However, I want to make sure that we remember that everyone is an individual and everyone is unique and we all have differences. Each person has their own history. Each person has their own experiences. All of this makes us all unique. God is an artist and very creative. He has created us all so individually and so differently.

We are also the sum total of what all of our ancestors thought and did, and our own experiences and decisions. Our ancestors were individuals that thought and behaved in certain ways, and the Bible says this:

Exodus 34:7b *Visiting the iniquity of the fathers upon the children, and upon the children's children, unto the third and to the fourth generation.*

What your ancestors thought and did has the potential to affect you today. It can affect you negatively with curses or it can affect you positively with blessings. We can hear this called familiar spirits. These familiar spirits or ways or thinking, believing and behaving can come down from generation to generation.

God's word tells us this also:

Deuteronomy 7:9 *Know therefore that the LORD thy God, he is God, the faithful God, which keepeth covenant and mercy with them that love him and keep his commandments to a thousand generations;*

When we are hearers and doers of the word, our generations will be blessed. When you came into the world, you came with your own set of familiar spirits or patterns of thinking and behaving that came from your ancestors.

Everyone has a different experience growing up and everyone has different experiences as adults. Though we all tribulate, some people may seem to have more problems or tribulations than others do. It depends on how we have reacted to our tribulations that will determine how we think and believe and feel and behave. We have to look at each individual and deal with their own set of individual circumstances in order to accurately determine what thoughts and behaviors they have that don't line up with God and His word.

Everyone is very different from everyone else. We are all people. We all created beings. We have the same Father in heaven, who created us, but we are all very unique and individual in our creation and in our lives. We all have our own unique histories.

I want to reiterate that although the articles and studies that we read are important and they show the truth of the mind and body connection, we also have to remember that these studies do not understand God and His word. These studies do not look at these personality traits through Godly eyes. They don't take God and His word into account. God and His word can change our lives.

There is much more that we have to look at when we look at how people think and behave when we take God and His word into account. We do have a starting place which is God's word. We can compare our thoughts and behaviors to God and His word and then we can discern where Satan and his kingdom might have influenced us.

That is what my goal is in this book. We have to look at the thoughts and behaviors of the individual person that has a disease process in their body and help them to recognize when they are thinking and behaving in ways that do not line up with God and His word.

I want to make it clear that it is important to look at each individual person and their unique history to be able to help them to see what is happening to them.

Although, it can be helpful to look at the roots from A More Excellent Way or the character and personality traits that the medical community has described that seem to be present in people who have been diagnosed with cancer, we ultimately have to look at each person individually.

— CHAPTER THREE —

The Great Exchange

We, as ministers of the gospel, can then help people to admit and recognize what thoughts and behaviors that they have that don't line up with God and His word. We can help them to purpose in their hearts to quit these issues, and exchange them with new ways of thinking and behaving that do line up with God and His word.

I call this the GREAT EXCHANGE. We exchange our old ways of thinking that are conducive to sickness and disease and we put in their place new ways of thinking that come from God and His word and lead us into health and wholeness.

Don't forget, each person is so very unique. God is very creative. Each of us has been created to be unique by God. We all have different gifts and talents. We all have different ancestors who made their own decisions and had their own experiences. We also, have had our own unique and different experiences in our own lives.

This information leads us to dealing with each person's set of circumstances individually.

Individual Personality Traits

Let's begin to more closely examine the personality traits that seem to be present in people who have diseases or specifically cancer. The first personality trait that I would like to address is that these people can be fabricating a personality. They can essentially be imposters or living a lie.

Living a Lie

Actually, the most prevalent issue that I see in this disease profile for cancer is that the person actually lives a lie.

They don't tell the truth about themselves or how they really think or feel about things. They can fabricate their personality in order to please others and avoid conflict. They can be denying, ignoring, repressing or suppressing their real thoughts, feelings and emotions. Those who fail to acknowledge their desperation may be at higher risk.

Working with breast-cancer patients, Mogens Jensen of the Yale psychology department showed that 'defensive-repressors' die faster than patients with a more realistic outlook. These are the smiling ones who don't acknowledge their desperation, who say, 'I'm fine,' even though you know they have cancer, their spouses have run off, their children are drug addicts, and the house just burned down. Jensen feels this behavior 'disregulates' and exhausts the immune system because it is confused by the mixed messages[33]."

One of the things that stands out about this person is that they act as if nothing is wrong. They can be having the worst day of their lives, but they will have a smile on their face. If you ask them if they have any problems, they deny that anything is really wrong. You know that they have a disease or they just lost their job or they have chronic pain or they have just lost their house, but they are just not saying anything about it. This is **DENIAL**.

An acronym for denial is: **D**on't **E**ven **N**o **I A**m **L**ying. (Note: The originator of this acronym used the word NO but it is really the word KNOW. They sound the same! And they create an easy acronym to remember.)

Being in denial is really lying. You are lying to yourself and to God and to other people. You don't even know that you are lying or not telling yourself, God or other people the truth that is in your heart.

I call this the "speedy Christian." They say things like: "Oh I am healed," and they zoom off. "Nothing is wrong with me, I have faith." " I know God has healed me. I have nothing wrong with me."

Yet, the truth is that they are sick, really sick. They are not facing the truth about their situation.

They mistakenly think that if they don't talk about their issues, if they don't feel their feelings, then they are following God and His word. People can think that if they just don't talk about their issues, that they have gone away. They think that this behavior will lead to healing. They think that they can just name what they want and then have it. This kind of thinking has been called "NAME IT AND CLAIM IT." I call it lying about it and depending on God to do what you want Him to do without taking responsibility for our own problems or sin issues.

These people can be bald from all of the drugs that they take for their disease. They are lonely, miserable and frightened and they have no REAL hope or vision for their future. They are speeding and zooming right past the real issues in their lives.

You can ask them if they have had any side effects from the drugs that the doctors have given them and they can say, "I got sick, could not eat or sleep, I had pain and I lost my hair."

But they have denied that anything has been wrong in their lives. They don't face the truth or talk about the truth or deal with the truth with God. They are living a lie. They speed right past the truth. They go right past their feelings.

Here is a scripture where God tells us what can happen if we go right past our feelings and we don't face what is really in our hearts, minds and lives.

Ephesians 4:17-19 *[17]This I say therefore, and testify in the Lord, that ye henceforth walk not as other Gentiles walk, in the vanity of their mind, [18]Having the understanding darkened, being alienated from the life of God through the ignorance that is in them, because of the blindness of their heart: [19]Who being past feeling have given themselves over unto lasciviousness, to work all uncleanness with greediness.*

Ask yourself this question: Are you past feeling? Are you leaning on your own understanding? Are you listening to the dark thoughts that come into your mind that come from Satan and his kingdom? Are you perishing for lack of knowledge or ignorance? Do you have veils over your eyes and ears? Are you putting on blinders? Are you speeding right past your true thoughts and feelings?

Are You in Denial?

We can have spiritual and emotional and behavioral roots to our diseases and we can be in denial of our true problems or sin issues. We don't even know that they we are lying. D-E-N-I-A-L.

People can deny that there is a problem, they can refuse to address their problems and they lie to themselves and to God and to other people. We can be past feeling and into all kinds of sin. The result is that we can seem so very nice, we can have forced smiles, and we can be very polite when we are really displaying insincere or inauthentic behavior.

These people are not genuine in their behavior. They are fabricating their personality and their responses. They are lying. They are denying, repressing or suppressing their real feelings and thoughts. They can be manipulating everyone around them so that they don't have to face the truth. They want to present an untrue picture of themselves. The truth can feel just too difficult to face or to deal with or to admit. They just don't want to cause conflict or have to have difficult interactions or conversations.

A lot of time you can see that they will laugh or smile inappropriately or at the wrong times. They can be fabricating their personality to be accepted and loved. The real truth is that they think that they can't tell the truth or they think, "If I tell the truth, there will be consequences or strife or conflict or I can be rejected. I don't want to rock the boat." They can think that they have too much to lose if they tell the truth.

They want to avoid conflict or any difficult feelings at all costs. They may just not know how to deal with conflict. They don't have the skills or assurance to deal with conflict and they can feel that they are inadequate or unable to cope with the consequences of any conflict. They don't express their true emotions or what they are truly thinking. They don't want to deal with controversial issues because they want to continue to have some kind of control in their lives. Controversial issues are unpredictable and that makes them very uncomfortable.

Here are some examples of people who don't tell the truth about what is happening in their lives:

1. A woman who stays married to a man who physically abuses her. The woman feels that she can't really tell the truth because she thinks that she can't leave the situation because she has no money and no way to support herself. She may think that if she leaves, no one else will want to be with her and she will be alone all of her life. She has poor self esteem and no vision for herself for the future. She can become codependent with her husband's sin of abuse she remains a victim and the situation never changes.

2. People can think that they should not tell the truth because even if they did tell the truth, there would be no change in the situation that they are in. They can believe that if they tell the truth they would be suffering the consequences of telling the truth with no hope for change.

3. People won't tell the truth because they think that they can't handle facing the truth. The truth can feel so overwhelming and so painful that they think that it would be too much to bear. They can end up denying and suppressing the truth and in the end, making themselves sick.

4. People don't want to tell the truth because they don't want to hurt the people that love them. They think that they are protecting other people. They think that they are protecting their relationship with the other person.

5. People don't want to tell the truth because they want to avoid arguments and debates and conflict. They think that they are protecting themselves and their lives and relationships.

6. Another reason that people lie is because of fear. They fear that the truth would not get them what they want. The bottom line is that people fear that if they tell the truth, they will not get what they want, anyway.

7. Sometimes people don't want to tell the truth because they feel that if they admit what they really think and feel, they will be either rejected or ridiculed or abandoned. They may think that others will make fun of them or lose respect for them.

8. Finally, people don't tell the truth because they are programmed to fabricate and lie. It is a habit for them and a stronghold in their

lives. It can be a familiar spirit that came down through their family line and they don't even know that they are fabricating. This is a way of life for them.

These are just a few of the reasons that people deny the truth or fail to tell it if, in fact, they do know the truth.

What do we notice in all of these reasons not to tell the truth? It is a selfishness, a self focus, it is the ME ME ME ME syndrome. Everything is all about me. It is "EVERYTHING I." Everything is focused on me.

I want to tell a short story here about "EVERYTHING I." Many years ago, when I was sick, I met a woman that had gotten well from the incurable (re: stated by the doctors to be incurable) disease that I had. This woman told me that she had been sick with the same disease. The disease was called Environmental Illness. The acronym for this disease is EI. She told me that she had been healed of the disease. I asked her how she got healed. She said that she had a dream and in her dream Jesus held up a sign to her. The sign said "EI" (EVERYTHING I). She said that she realized that she was self focused and selfish and into self-pity. She said she repented to God and she and God changed everything and she got well.

I never forgot her story. It impacted my life.

When we are selfish and self-focused, we can be living with the attitude that everything is about me. We can feel entitled to having everything go our own way and that breeds disappointment. If we don't deal with our disappointment with God, disappointment can breed sorrow and lots of anger.

Another one of the biggest reasons that people don't tell the truth is that they just don't know the truth of how they feel. They don't even know how to tell how or what they are truly feeling. Sometimes people can feel NUMB.

Sometimes we just don't know the truth!

Again, the acronym for denial is that I **d**on't **e**ven "**n**o" that **I a**m **l**ying.

Let me give you some examples:

You have an interaction with someone that you don't feel comfortable with and yet you smile and act as if you are just fine. You are not admitting the truth to yourself. You feel uncomfortable, but you just ignore it. This causes stress and anxiety and conflict in your heart and mind and this manifests in your physical body.

An example of this in my own life is that I was attending a class. I was not really comfortable with what the people were saying, but I just went back time after time. I finally realized and admitted the truth to myself. I was uncomfortable and I did not have to return to the class.

It is not that you have to say something to the other person, but at the very least, you should tell the truth to yourself and God. Ignoring and denying what you feel can affect your body. Next time that you are uncomfortable in an interaction, stop and take notice how your body feels. What are you really feeling and thinking? You may find that your true feelings are painful or even terrifying. However, if we allow ourselves to acknowledge our true thoughts and feelings, we can deal with them in a Godly way and we don't have to have consequences in our bodies. Feelings are just feelings, thoughts are just thoughts, it is our decision if we listen to them or act on them.

When I began to do this, I noticed that I had subtle changes and feelings in my body that I ignored because I was so used to them.

But these feelings are trying to tell us something. They may be confusing or painful, but they can also lead us to the roots of our issues and then our healing. They can affect our bodies if we don't deal with our issues with God and resolve them.

I recently spoke with a woman whose daughter has cancer, I asked her how her daughter was. She said, "Oh, she is just fine." I was shocked. The daughter had just found out that she had a fast growing cancer and the mother was not showing any emotion. She continued on to say, "She just went to Texas to a hospital that specializes in the kind of cancer that she has." She continued to say, "She was smiling and happy when I saw her. She seems fine and happy. I am sure that she will be fine."

I thought as I heard this I could not find a better example of denial. Again, remember the acronym for denial: I don't even "no" I am lying. I asked the woman "Do you think that she is really okay with this?" And she said, "Maybe she was putting on a false front."

Putting on a "false front" is exactly what was probably happening. It would be common sense to know that this person had other feelings that she was not sharing or expressing or acknowledging.

Inherited Patterns of Familiar Spirits

Another thing that the Bible says Exodus 20:5 and Deuteronomy 5:9 *"I the Lord thy God am a jealous God, visiting the iniquity of the fathers upon the children unto the third and fourth generation of them that hate me."*

What is this telling us? The thoughts and behaviors that our parents do … we can also do.

I have found that the behaviors that the parents do, the children also do, in some way or another. It does not have to be in the same exact way, but in general, if I know that a parent has a particular behavior pattern, I look for that same behavior pattern in the child. More often than not, I will find it in the child's life. It manifests in some way or another.

So, I can extrapolate in this example situation that if the mother has such great denial in her personality, we may also find it in the daughter.

Another example of this is if a father is angry and violent in his behavior you will see it in the son in one way or another.

When unhealthy behavior patterns are modeled to children by their parents, you can find the behavior pattern in the children. It can be manifesting in a different way, but if you look you will find that the person has a familiar spirit that has been passed down from their parents and they generally don't even know it.

People can be taught to live in denial. They just don't face the truth because it is can seem so difficult to face. The way to change this is to accept God into our lives and begin to renew our minds and wash with the water of the word. Consequently we can change the way that we think and behave.

Accepting God into our lives is just our first step towards a relationship with God. Our goal is to be changed and transformed into the image of Christ. We want to think and behave like Jesus would have and did while He was on this planet. This takes time and commitment and study.

The best example of this is something that I see all of the time. When someone has a problem in a relationship, for example in their marriage or a close friendship, they can't be honest about their feelings for fear of causing problems or afraid of the other person's reactions. As a result, they end up manipulating the situation because they know that if they say or express how they really feel the other person might reject them. They just choose to deny their problems. They don't face the truth nor talk about the truth of the situation.

This is lying. It is living a lie. It is not being honest with yourself or with the other person or with God. It is living in denial and ignoring or suppressing or repressing the truth. This is why it's manipulative: Causing others to "believe" a lie that everything is alright.

Another example can be that something happens that you don't like and it makes you angry or really uncomfortable or it actually hurts your feelings and you may tell yourself, "Nothing is the matter, I am feeling this, but feelings don't matter any way. I can make this look all okay—I won't feel it. If I ignore this, maybe it will go away. I won't rock the boat."

Another example of this can be perhaps you are in a job or a relationship that is not fulfilling or right for you, and yet you keep trying to make it work by living within the rules of the relationship. You are unwilling to feel your true feelings for fear that it may be too overwhelming to deal with. These are just some examples that show us how people can say one thing and be thinking and feeling something very different.

I have an example of this that I admitted to myself recently. I had a relationship with a friend that had a lot of good qualities and I liked a lot of things about her. But every time we got together she said and did things that were controlling, manipulative and sarcastic. She did not realize that she was doing this, but for my part, I never said anything.

I was in denial and I accepted this behavior so that I could remain friends with her. I knew that if I said anything there would be some conflict. I never felt comfortable when I was with her, I always felt anxious. I would not feel comfortable after every interaction with her. I was allowing myself to be victimized and co-dependent, and yet I let it continue out of fear of loss and rejection.

This type of denial is just lying. I was lying to myself and I was not doing her any favors either. Because I was not being honest about the issues in the relationship, I was lying to my friend also. She thought that everything was okay between us. I was lying to myself and to her and to God. I was not in a relationship that was healthy for me. I was subjecting myself to being hurt by my reactions to her behavior.

Lying to yourself can sap your energy level when you ignore what is really going on in your life. Lying to yourself, to God and to others can affect your immune system.

It is bad for our health when we don't deal with the truth in our lives.

Here is a story that shows us how we can get healed when we face the truth.

Cynthia Rose Young Schlosser, October 2002, edited & published by Healing Cancer Naturally with special permission of the author.

Many years ago my grandmother on my father's side was in a (bad) similar position. Her cancer had spread everywhere and she was given only 3 to 6 months to live. Knowing her end was near, she found the courage to stand up to my grandfather, who was a very controlling and stern man, and she refused to let him control her any longer. [My grandfather had prohibited music and dancing, and when she learned she was going to die, she defied him, saying that he couldn't tell a dying woman what to do.] They wanted to take off her leg to extend her life. She told them that if she only had less than a year to live, that she wanted her leg during that time, and she walked out of the doctor's office, went to Rich's and bought a record player and lots of Elvis Presley records and went home and danced and danced—something he had strictly forbidden. She went to the old folks home and played hymns for them on their old piano, another thing that had been forbidden. My grandmother loved Elvis so much.

Well, she just got better and better and better. She got completely well! It all went into remission. She outlived all my other grandparents. She lived for 20 more years, dying finally of a heart attack in the night. I remember once when she took a Greyhound bus many miles to visit us just to walk me to the record store (a long walk I might add) to buy me an Elvis record. What a beautiful grandmother she was! She taught me about miracles by her own beautiful example[34]. *Cynthia Rose's grandmother spontaneously healed of terminal cancer by being true to herself.*

Even if we don't have a disease in our bodies or in our minds we may all see some of these issues in our own lives. We may see that we are not being completely honest with ourselves and with God.

If there is one thing that I would say is number one on the list to getting well—it would be to tell the truth to yourself and God and in your relationships. Deal with the truth in a Godly way.

Disease Prevention

It is always beneficial to look at our behaviors and judge ourselves. God says this in the word:

1 Corinthians 11:31 *For if we would judge ourselves, we should not be judged.*

If we judge ourselves; if we are being washed with the water of the word and we are renewing our minds, then we are going to be able to discern and to see the things in our lives that don't line up with God and His word. We can compare our thoughts and behaviors with God and His word, and then we can see where we are not lining up with Him.

We are judging ourselves and our thoughts and our own actions. If we judge ourselves and we then recognize and admit our sins, we can purpose in our hearts to quit our sins and exchange them with Godly thoughts and behaviors from the Bible.

We are now practicing disease prevention! We are judging ourselves so that God does not have to judge us.

In other words we are choosing to be hearers and doers of the word. What a blessing it is to be able to recognize our own sins and then exchange them with the word of God. So, by exposing the devil and his thoughts and his behaviors and exchanging them with thoughts and behaviors that come from God and His word, we can practice disease prevention. Even though I am discussing cancer in this book, we can all learn a lot about things that we may be doing in our own lives. These issues or behaviors can be applied to any disease.

No matter what our sin issues are, we can purpose in our hearts to work with God to change these issues so that they are lining up with God and His word.

God tells us this in:

Deuteronmoy 28:2 *And all these blessings shall come on thee, and overtake thee, if thou shalt hearken unto the voice of the LORD thy God.*

We want the blessings that God has for us to overtake us!

The words "come on thee and overtake thee" tell us that these blessings will come into our lives, they will follow us and there will be nothing that we can do to stop them. They will overtake us. That sounds awesome to me!

We have to remember our part in this scripture. We have to harken to the voice of God, and then the blessings will overtake us. This is a promise from God. How do we put this into action? How do we harken to the voice of the Lord?

Well, when we are discussing cancer, some of the characteristics that can alert you to a Type C ("Cancer") personality can be that the person seems to be saying that everything is fine and they are smiling, but they are really not telling the truth. They are having problems and they are in denial about them. They are not facing the truth.

Remember that we said that the acronym for denial is: "**D**on't **E**ven "**N**o" that **I A**m **L**ying?"

Remember what the articles and the studies say: "The coping style of Type C personalities, i.e. excessive denial, avoidance, suppression and repression of emotions, appears to weaken natural resistance to carcinogenic influences."

The opposite of this would be if we face the truth and tell the truth we will be strengthening our immune systems. This is harkening to the voice of the Lord. We are telling the truth.

So, harkening to the voice of the Lord can be being honest and transparent and telling the truth to God, ourselves and to others.

Proverbs 10:18 *He that hideth hatred with lying lips, and he that uttereth a slander, is a fool.*

This scripture says it all. When you are angry it can eventually lead to hatred. When you hide your hatred and then you gossip or murder others with your tongue or in your heart or with your actions or your hands, the Bible says that you are a fool. God is telling us that it is foolish to lie about how you really feel. It is foolish to lie or to live in denial. You can't work anything out with God or anyone else if you don't tell the truth or face the truth.

Here is another scripture that speaks directly to the problem:

Proverbs 12:22 *Lying lips are abomination to the LORD: but they that deal truly are his delight.*

This lets us know that the Lord finds lying an abomination or disgusting, but when we deal with things honestly and truly, He is delighted.

God wants us to be honest in our relationships. He wants us to be faithful and dependable. We have to tell the truth. We can't ignore or close our eyes to what is really happening in our lives, if we do, we are liars.

We have to acknowledge our feelings. It does not mean that we have to act on our feelings or that our feelings are emergencies or that our feelings are right. However, we have to acknowledge them and then work them out in a Godly way.

Denying our feelings, or repressing or suppressing our feelings is not healthy. We have to face what we are feeling and then decide to work out our feelings in a Godly way. Remember this scripture:

Ephesians 4:26 *Be ye angry, and sin not.*

It is not a sin to be angry or to have thoughts or emotions or feelings. We just have to deal with them in a Godly manner. We don't want to sin just because we have a feeling.

We can cast out devils, we can cast down our thoughts, but we have to deal with our feelings. We can't cast out our feelings as if they were devils, we have to deal with them with God and decide to act in Godly ways.

Our feelings do not have to be telling us the truth. FEELINGS can be liars. Always remember that we can get our thoughts from God, ourselves or Satan and his kingdom. We have to check out everything we think or feel. For example, if you are feeling guilty, that does not necessarily mean that you are guilty. If you are feeling like you want to hurt someone else, you don't have to be in agreement with that feeling. Feelings tell us what is going on in our thoughts. Our feelings come out of what we believe to be true. When all the time, we can believe lies that come from Satan and his kingdom.

If we have thoughts that say that we are guilty and we get into agreement with them and we think that we are guilty, then we can have feelings of guilt and condemnation. These feelings are the fruit of the thoughts or the beliefs that are telling us that we are guilty. These original thoughts could be coming from Satan!

If we are feeling guilty, then all sorts of other feelings can start to hang around. We can blame ourselves and begin to let unloving spirits or self hatred come into our lives. We can allow an evil spirit of accusation to speak to us.

Feelings are not meant to be acted upon or believed just because we have them. Feelings are meant to help tell us that something may be wrong and that we should address the issue. Feelings should not be ignored, denied, suppressed or repressed, but we should strive to properly interpret what they are trying to tell us.

For example: if you feel guilty, the devil might have told you to think, "Oh, I am guilty. It is all my fault. I can never fix this. I made such a big mistake. I am so angry with myself. I hate myself. I can't do anything right. Nothing can ever change or get better."

If you know God and His word, you will know that all of this is just lies.

Jeremiah 29:11 *For I know the thoughts that I think toward you, saith the LORD, thoughts of peace, and not of evil, to give you an expected end [a future and a hope].*

All of the negativity in your mind is not coming from God. God has good plans for us so these thoughts have to be coming from Satan who wants you to think and feel badly and hopeless and helpless.

You have to know the word of God to know that you are hearing a thought that does not come from God. You have to say, "No! That thought is just the devil and I am having feelings that come from that thought. I don't have to listen to you, Satan."

You then have to look at the issue and deal with the truth of your thoughts and feelings with God.

For example, if you recognized that you were feeling guilty, you can deal with the issue with God. You can cast down the thought and you can cast out the devil who wants you to feel guilty. You can tell God all about what you are feeling. You can remind Satan that God forgives us when we take responsibility and have a repentant heart. We have choices. One choice is that we can continue to agree with the devil and we can continue to let the devil beat us up about our past mistakes.

Or, we can decide that we need to get to the root of the problem and address it with God's Word. What does God's Word say about our guilt?

It tells us that if we confess our sin and repent and purpose in our hearts to quit the sin, we are forgiven and cleansed of whatever kind of unrighteousness or sin that we've committed.

We can admit our sin, quit our sin and exchange the wrong thoughts and beliefs with the right ones from God's word. When we choose to confess our sins and repent to God and purpose in our hearts to quit our sins, then our feelings will change also.

Our feelings can be the fruit of our thoughts and beliefs. Even if we did make a mistake in the past, the word says that when we admit our sins and quit them and exchange them for the word of truth with a truly repentant heart, God forgives us our sins.

Remember, our feelings are just the fruit of our thoughts and beliefs. Our feelings can be a great revealer of what we are really thinking and believing under the surface. Our feelings can tell us a lot about what is truly in our hearts and minds. Remember this important point: Our thoughts can come from God or Satan or from our own experiences and decisions.

Change Your Thinking

The truth is that we have to change our thinking to God's way of thinking. The gospel—the Good News about Jesus Christ and the Kingdom of God —is all about changing our thinking. Changing our thinking will lead to a change in our feelings and doings.

We have to believe that we can express the truth about how we feel about things to ourselves and to God and to other people. You have to be willing to be honest in all of your relationships. We have to face the truth no matter how difficult it can seem. God is all about the truth and change and transformation and behavior modification.

The gospel is all about behavior modification!

James 1:22 *But be ye doers of the word, and not hearers only, deceiving your own selves.*

Being a doer of the word is all about behavior modification. When we change our behavior and we tell the truth, we have the opportunity to be honest with God and with ourselves and with other people. When we face the truth, we then have the opportunity to change things in our lives.

When we deny the truth, we are not being honest, we are fabricating and we are lying. We are deceiving ourselves. We are lying to ourselves. And we are lying to other people and more importantly, we are lying to God. We can't change what we don't admit!

When we are lying to ourselves, we are letting the devil lie to us and we are believing his lies. Ultimately, when we do that we are listening to Satan and his kingdom.

One of the biggest problems that we have is that we believe lies. We believe the thoughts that come into our minds. We think that they are our own and we let them influence our lives.

We have to remember that the thoughts that come into our minds can come from one of three places. They can come from God, from Satan and his kingdom or from our own minds, experiences and decisions that we have made. The only thoughts that we should be listening to are thoughts that line up with God and His word. Satan and his Kingdom are going to be telling us lies. Look at this scripture:

> **John 8:44** (Christ speaking to evil religious leaders) *Ye are of your father the devil, and the lusts of your father ye will do. He was a murderer from the beginning, and abode not in the truth, because there is no truth in him. When he speaketh a lie, he speaketh of his own: for he is a liar, and the father of it.*

Satan is the father of lies and he wants us to believe all of his lies. Just because you have a thought, it does not mean that you have to get into agreement with it and continue to entertain it. As a matter of fact, the Bible tells us to watch all of our thoughts and to get rid of them if they don't agree with God and His word.

> **2 Corinthians 10:5** *Casting down imaginations, and every high thing that exalteth itself against the knowledge of God, and bringing into captivity every thought to the obedience of Christ.*

In other words, we can't and should not just let our thoughts run wildly through our minds; we have to watch our thoughts. If they don't agree with God and His word, we cast them down. We decide not to think them and we replace them with thoughts that agree with God and His word.

In order to know what Satan's lies are, we have to be renewing our minds with God's word all of the time.

Romans 12:2 *And be not conformed to this world: but be ye transformed by the renewing of your mind, that ye may prove what is that good, and acceptable, and perfect, will of God.*

We want to wash our minds clean from the lies of Satan and replace the lies with the truth of God.

Ephesians 5:26 *That he might sanctify and cleanse it with the washing of water by the word.*

Just like water will wash our bodies clean, so will the words in the Bible wash our minds clean of wrong thoughts and beliefs.

John 8:32 *And ye shall know the truth, and the truth shall make you free.*

The truth of God represents health and healing to our bodies and to our minds.

People Pleasers

Another example of lying and being in denial is a behavior pattern which can be referred to as "people pleasers." In one of the articles and studies that we looked at; we saw that one of the behavior patterns that the Type C personality has is this: "A deep desire to make others happy, often at their own expense (people pleasers) or being pathologically nice."

What does it mean to be a people pleaser?

If you have a "People pleaser behavior pattern", you may try to be someone whom other people want you to be. You may fabricate your personality so that it pleases whomever you are with. You can be like a chameleon, ever changing who you are to be able to satisfy other people. Your main goal may be to agree with other people so that you will be accepted and liked. You want to fit in. Your goal is to be accepted and not rejected. You may not be aware that you are doing this, (remember our old friend denial), but you may find yourself trying to please others in order to avoid reactions that you are afraid of. Your fears may come from wanting others to like you so that they will not abandon or reject you. You can be trying to avoid conflict.

You are actually being motivated by a spirit of fear. You can be trying to control situations so that you can feel safe and not have to "rock the boat." You can also be motivated by wanting to get your self esteem and self worth from how others feel about you.

When you are a people pleaser, if someone is mad at you, it can ruin your whole day or whole week or even your whole life. You can base your happiness, peace, self worth and self esteem on what other people think about you.

In other words, if we are people pleasers, we are trying to stay safe and comfortable, and we are trying to feel good about ourselves because of what other people think about us. We see ourselves as worthy because of other people's opinions of us.

In reality, doing something for someone out of the wrong motive is actually manipulation and control. It amounts to divination and witchcraft. Here are several examples of some behaviors that come from people pleasers and how they think and behave.

An example could be that someone whom you have a relationship with tells us that you don't spend enough time with them. You immediately feel badly and you want to make sure that you figure out how to give this person the time that they want. You feel conflicted, guilty and you get stressed and anxious.

The problem is that your goal is to satisfy the other person's desires so that they are not angry with you. You want them to accept you and to be pleased with what you do. Behind your desire to satisfy them is your own fear of man and abandonment, rejection and conflict. You want to conform or satisfy their demands to avoid conflict.

What could you do instead? The mature thing to do would be to decide if the other person's demands are reasonable for you. You have to decide if the person is just controlling and demanding something that you cannot give or do not want to give.

Communication

You can ask yourself some questions. Do you have more time to spend with this person; is the person's evaluation of the situation the same as yours? There is a lot of thinking and communicating that can go into your decision. You have to know what the real issue is in the relationship.

But, if you are a people pleaser your main thought is "how can I please this person? How can I make sure that this person will not be angry with me? I must make sure that I satisfy this person's request so that I am not rejected or abandoned. I have to make sure that there is no conflict. I have to be nice and satisfy this person."

However, ask yourself what is really going on in your heart and mind and in your emotions? That is important to know. If you end up doing things to please other people and you have anger simmering in your heart, this leads to conflict within yourself and anxiety and eventually disease.

The truth is that there is a difference between people pleasing and doing things unto the Lord. When we do things unto the Lord—or we do things because we are serving the Lord—our decisions come out of wanting to please Him. We want to do what the Lord would have us do. We know that if we follow God and His word and His ways, He will bless us.

When we do things because we are people pleasing we are in denial. We don't even know we are lying. We are doing things so that we can stop our own fear. We are not being honest or looking for the honest and true issues in our lives.

We are simply in idolatry to ourselves. We want things to go our own way, we are trying to control our lives and other people. We are actually manipulating other people and this amounts to witchcraft.

Colossians 3:23 *And whatsoever ye do, do it heartily, as to the Lord, and not unto men.*

Colossians 3:17 *And whatever you do in word or deed, do all in the name of the Lord Jesus, giving thanks to God the Father through Him.*

"Whatever" in this scripture refers to all that we do or everything that we say. Paul wrote that whatever we do, whether it is what we say or we do, we are to do it in the name of Jesus.

If we are truly doing things and saying things in the name of Jesus, and we are doing and saying things unto the Lord, it would be difficult to justify doing or saying things that we would not say or do if Jesus were on the planet and watching us. It would be hard to justify continuing in thought and behaviors that absolutely did not come from God and His word.

For example: If you were gossiping would you be able to say, "I am doing this unto the Lord?" If you were stealing would you be able to say, "I am doing this in the name of the Lord?" If you are lying or manipulating or trying to control a situation or a person, would you be able to say, "I am doing this in the name of the Lord?" It would be as if when you were looking at pornography you would say "In the name of Jesus, I am looking at this pornography." You would immediately know that this was not going to please the Lord. It was not an activity that the Lord condones.

The Bible tells us how to behave and think. We can apply the basic principles in the Bible to just about every situation that we get into on this planet. Anything you want to do that you cannot do "as unto the Lord," obviously is something you should <u>not</u> do. At the very least, you should really think about what you are doing.

This Scripture answers questions like, "Can I, in Jesus' name, as a Christian, smoke pot or smoke cigarettes, or get drunk, or shoot up with heroin, or get involved in an illicit sexual situation or manipulate someone to get what I want? Can I stay angry and hold grudges and seek revenge against someone?"

The question to ask yourself is this, "Can you do those things in the name of Jesus?" "Am I trying to please people or am I trying to please God?"

This is powerful. If we think about this in our daily lives or in our relationships, we can answer a lot of our own questions.

Another example of being a people pleaser can be is if someone says something to you that bothers you, annoys you or hurts you, you feel "funny" right away. You are affected by what the person says. Instead of clarifying what you heard the person say to you, you just change the subject or you make believe nothing was said or done that caused you to be concerned. You don't feel comfortable saying anything because you don't want to cause a conflict.

You want to make sure that the person likes you. You never really clarify the situation or deal with it honestly. The thought of being honest is actually terrifying to you.

This affects your relationships with other people and with yourself. The fear of man and fear of rejection and fear of abandonment will keep you stuck.

When we want to please others so that they don't hurt us by abandoning us or rejecting us or arguing with us, we can have a hard time saying "NO" or setting limits or having healthy boundaries with other people. We want to avoid conflict and we want other people's approval. We don't want others to disapprove of us.

We can be "approval junkies."

If someone asks us for something, we have a hard time not giving it. We just can't say no. We can be addicted to other people's approval of us. We just want to be accepted and loved. We want other people's approval so that we can feel "okay."

When you are a people pleaser, you can have trouble expressing your own feelings, desires or opinions.

You may not even know what you want or what you believe because it might be different from someone you want to please. You may end up making yourself think and feel what other people are thinking and feeling, because any difference is threatening. You don't want to rock the boat or make someone angry with you.

We can be so afraid of conflict and so afraid of doing things that other people don't like, that we can be in denial and we can be living a life filled with lies that we are not even aware of.

You may become confused and not really know what you are feeling or thinking or desiring because your goal is that you want to please the other person.

The problem with this is that you are doing things for the wrong reasons. You don't really want to do what you are being asked to do. Or maybe you really can't do what you are being asked to do, or you really should not do what you are being asked to do. However, you do it anyway so that the person will approve of you and not reject you. That is when resentment may start because you are doing what you don't want to do. The devil will influence you to continue to feel resentment which can graduate to holding a grudge and to wanting to retaliate in some way against the person.

You are now allowing the principality of bitterness to have access to your life. At some point, you can begin to retaliate or take revenge. This might come in the form of being passive-aggressive or saying something sarcastic or making fun of the person or giving the person the silent treatment. Another option can be that you can go to the other extreme and explode in rage and violence. The person you were pleasing doesn't know what hit them. They thought you were totally happy going along with them, and all of a sudden, you are acting differently.

You feel controlled and manipulated; and your needs are being ignored. You may feel as if you can't take it anymore. You are lying to yourself and to God and to the other person.

You are simmering below the surface. You have not dealt with the true issues with God. You have let the sun go down on your anger and it has been simmering. What we have to understand is that this simmering is harmful to your health. It is bitterness and it is holding a record of wrongs.

You have been lying and you have not had Godly motivations.

God does tell us to serve others and to love others and to prefer others, but He also tells us to love ourselves and to take care of our temples. He instructs us to tell the truth.

If we are in denial, we are not telling the truth. Here are some things that we may think when we are trying to please people. These are examples of some irrational beliefs of people with the people-pleasing personality traits:

- I must always do what others want of me.
- I must always put others before me.
- I must never say "No" to anyone.
- I must be liked by everyone.
- I must do nothing to upset others.
- I must work harder to make things better for others.
- They would never like me if they knew the truth about me.
- I must be careful in my decision making so as not to upset anyone.
- I can never do enough to please them.
- I am responsible for other peoples' happiness.
- How other people respond to me is crucial.
- The harder I work for them, the more they will appreciate me.

- If they don't like me, I'm no good!
- If they don't like me, I can't be at peace or be happy.
- Always put others first! Put yourself last. There is no task I won't do for you, large or small.
- People can only like you if you appear nice, pleasant, friendly, and cheerful to them. Your only role in life is giving to or helping others.
- If you are not successful, you are a loser and losers are ignored, unloved, and unwanted, rejected and abandoned.
- It's not who you are but what you do that counts.
- You must always be understanding and have an open mind with people who are hurting you or putting you down.
- If someone doesn't accept me, it must be that I'm not "good enough" to be accepted.
- No matter what I do, it never seems to be "good enough."
- I can do nothing right. I am worthless, useless, but I can't let others see this about me or they will reject me.

Here are a few examples of "should's" that the people pleaser expects of others:

- They should always like me because I try so hard to please them.
- They should never criticize me because I always try to live up to their expectations.
- They should never treat me unfairly because I am always so nice to them.
- I have done everything that they asked me to do, how can they be mean to me?

We can think that everyone has to like us or approve of us or we are not in peace.

However, the truth is that we don't have to be liked by everyone. We can't please everyone all of the time or even some of the time. Sometimes our own needs may have to take precedence over someone else's needs or desires.

Following is a list of feelings that we can see in people who want to people please. Feelings that can be associated with the people-pleasing personality traits. The following are taken from "People Pleasing Personality" by Jake Lawson[35]

- Fear of loss of approval
- Fear of rejection
- Fear of loss of personal identity
- Fear of loss of personal worth
- Denial of problems
- Self-denial or ignoring of personal rights
- Feeling lonely and isolated from others
- Avoid conflicts or fights at any cost
- Feeling not "good" enough
- Feeling undeserving
- Feeling inferior to others
- Concern about satisfying others' demands
- Insecurity about personal abilities, skills, or knowledge
- Compulsive need to please others
- Unhappy over not pleasing others
- Embarrassed by personal looks or behavior that displeases others
- Confusion about why it takes so much energy to please others
- Fear of not "doing best" for others' sake
- Fear of letting their friends and family down

- Fear of failure
- Fear of it being "found out" they are not as good as they appear to others
- Fear that others will recognize their failings
- Desire to run away to avoid the stress of always" needing to be "good"
- Exhaustion from always trying to be "perfect"
- Disappointment in not being able to make everyone happy
- Critical of how well they are doing in their personal lives
- Feel unappreciated or taken advantage of
- Feel taken for granted
- Feel like they are being treated like victims
- Feel like the martyr for others
- Fear of making a decision lest it be the wrong one
- Come unglued easily under pressure; unorganized

We should not let other people take advantage of us because we are listening to the spirit of fear tell us that if we don't please them, they will reject us.

This is another one of Satan's lies. Remember: listening to Satan's lies can set us up for sickness and disease.

Being a people pleaser is being a liar in the sense that we are not being honest with God, ourselves or to other people.

The bottom line is this: when we are people pleasers, we can be trying to please other people so that they will like us and approve of us. We don't want them to reject us. We can feel that we are always pressured to perform and fulfill other's expectations so that other people will accept us. We can think that we have to do and say what other people want us to do and say so that we gain their approval. We can think that we have to be perfect. We can base our self esteem on what other people think about us and what they think about what we do.

Trying to please other people can become so important to us that it can be like an addiction. It can be such a strong desire to us that it can influence our decisions about everyday life. We can become constantly addicted to pleasing people in order to feel okay or comfortable or in peace. We can think that if we don't do things and say things that please other people, they will reject or abandon us and those fears can lead us into having anxiety and no peace.

Do you have a pattern of being a people pleaser? Here are some self-diagnostic questions to consider:

1. Are you being truthful with yourself and with God and with other people?
2. Are you are saying and doing things to please others out of your own fear of rejection or fear of abandonment or fear of conflict?
3. Do you feel angry or irritated at yourself or the other person when you do or say things to please them?
4. Do you find yourself with anger or frustration simmering in your heart?

Instead of being truthful about our own desires, feelings and thoughts, we can develop a pattern of telling other people what we think that they want to hear so that we can be accepted by them.

Some things that we can think if we are people pleasers are:

1. I put others before myself, because it is the "good" and "right" thing to do.
2. If I told people what I really think they might be upset and stop liking me. They may reject me or abandon me or talk badly about me.
3. I spend a lot of energy being nice all the time, and I swallow any anger or the bad thoughts that I have.
4. I think a lot about how others might not like me or be disappointed with me.
5. Sometimes I feel drained meeting the needs of others, but I would never let that be known.

Here is A People-Pleaser Motto: *"I will be happy, pleasant, and liked by everyone."*

Some examples of being a people pleaser can also be like this: You can be in a conversation with someone where you agree with them with your words, but in reality in your heart you have a completely different opinion. For example, they say that they like Mexican food and you agree because you want them to like you. The truth is, you hate Mexican food but you say, "Oh yes, I love Mexican food, too. I will be glad to go to the restaurant you want to go to."

You just want to be accepted and so you just lie, lie, and lie some more. You are actually manipulating and controlling the other person so they will continue to like you. It is not a problem to compromise and do things that others like to do, the problem is doing things for the wrong reasons and then simmering inside because you resent having to do things or say things that you don't really agree with.

Another example can by that your friend asks you to do an errand for them. You really do not want to do it, you don't have the time to do it, but you say yes because you want them to like you. You want them to need you and you want them to depend on you. This can give you some security that they will still like you and accept you. The problem is that you do what was asked of you, but you have irritation and frustration simmering in your heart. This can lead you right into anger. You really needed the time to help yourself, but you were afraid to say no.

Another example can be that your boss asks you to work late and you say yes even though you have an important appointment after work. You want your boss to like you and you just can't bring yourself to say no.

Another example can be that your friend asks you to borrow your car. You absolutely want to say no, but you are afraid that they will be angry with you. You say yes, but you really—100%—wanted to say no.

You are lying and manipulating the other person to accept you and to like you and to not reject you. Most importantly, you are not taking care of yourself or seeking God. You are the one who suffers in these scenarios.

Another example can be that you have a relationship with someone and they don't treat you properly. They may be nasty or sarcastic to you, but you never say anything to them about it. You just don't want them to be angry with you. You don't want to cause conflict because they might not like you anymore. You feel hurt and angry when they say sarcastic things to you, but you just smile and let the anger simmer inside of your heart.

You are afraid that if you don't do or say what they want you to do or say, they may give you the silent treatment or they won't take your phone calls or they'll gossip about you to other people. They may have a party and they won't invite you. Or they may have a holiday gathering and they won't invite you. These very things are what you are trying to avoid.

I can go on and on with examples of this that I have seen in my own life and in other people's lives. I am sure that we all have examples of this, also. The truth is that we don't have to say yes when we really want to say no.

The truth is that you don't have to meet the demands and expectations of others if they are unreasonable, unrealistic or unfair. We don't have to say "yes" if we can't or we just don't want to do or say what the other person wants or needs.

We don't have to accept abuse because we are afraid of being rejected.

In summary, we don't have to always agree with what other people want us to say and do. We do, however, have to be honest and truthful with ourselves and with God.

When you can't be truthful, when you are performing to get love and your self esteem, the tension of doing this can wear you out.

People pleasing can literally stress you out! It can wear you out and leave you wiped out! It causes anxiety and conflict within us, which is ultimately the precursor to disease.

The bottom line is this: We can be saying yes when we really want to say no and we can be doing all of that for the wrong reasons. Doing things or saying things for these reasons is really manipulative and controlling and it is not honest. It is doing things for the wrong reasons.

Again, remember, don't say "yes" when you really want to or need to say "no." In order to have esteem or to be important or valuable, you may feel that you have to please other people. You may think that your self esteem comes from what others think of you, and that is a tough place to be.

People are just people, they can't be happy with everything that you do or say. We can't and won't agree with everything that others say and do. We are all created by God to be unique and different.

We are only people but we are all individuals and we have our own thoughts and desires and gifts and talents. We are all important. Where would the other parts of the body be without us?

1 Corinthians 12:14-20 *¹⁴For the body is not one member, but many. ¹⁵If the foot shall say, Because I am not the hand, I am not of the body; is it therefore not of the body? ¹⁶And if the ear shall*

say, Because I am not the eye, I am not of the body; is it therefore not of the body? ¹⁷If the whole body were an eye, where were the hearing? If the whole were hearing, where were the smelling? ¹⁸But now hath God set the members every one of them in the body, as it hath pleased him. ¹⁹And if they were all one member, where were the body? ²⁰But now are they many members, yet but one body.

We are all members of the body of Christ and we are members of our families and our communities and our state and our country. And ultimately we are all members of planet earth. At the same time we are all individuals and unique. We are all important to God. If we try and please others by not being honest with God or ourselves or others, we are liars and we are not telling the truth. The Bible is very clear about what God thinks about lying.

Let's look at a scripture we have talked about before:

Revelation 21:8 *But the fearful, and unbelieving, and the abominable, and murderers, and whore-mongers, and sorcerers, and idolaters, and all liars, shall have their part in the lake which burneth with fire and brimstone: which is the second death.*

Lying hurts us. When we lie to ourselves and God about what is really in our hearts and minds, it is allowing Satan access to our lives.

It is God that is the one that should give us our self esteem or what I call our God esteem. It is God who defines us and tells us who we are.

We are children of the most high God, we are the apple of His eye. He created us in our mother's womb. He loves us unconditionally and He has good plans for us.

Here are some scriptures that tell us all about these biblical truths:

Galatians 3:26 *For ye are all the children of God by faith in Christ Jesus.*

Deuteronomy 32:10 *He found him in a desert land, and in the waste howling wilderness; he led him about, he instructed him, he kept him as the apple of his eye.*

Psalm 139:13 *For thou hast possessed my reins: thou hast covered me in my mother's womb.*

Jeremiah 1:5 *Before I formed thee in the belly I knew thee; and before thou camest forth out of the womb I sanctified thee.*

Jeremiah 29:11 *For I know the thoughts that I think toward you, saith the LORD, thoughts of peace, and not of evil, to give you an expected end.*

Zephaniah 3:17 *The LORD thy God in the midst of thee is mighty; he will save, he will rejoice over thee with joy; he will rest in his love, he will joy over thee with singing.*

Ephesians 2:4-5 *But God, who is rich in mercy, for his great love wherewith he loved us, ⁵Even when we were dead in sins, hath quickened us together with Christ, (by grace ye are saved;).*

1 John 4:9-10 *⁹In this was manifested the love of God toward us, because that God sent his only begotten Son into the world, that we might live through him. ¹⁰Herein is love, not that we loved God, but that he loved us, and sent his Son to be the propitiation for our sins.*

1 John 3:1 *Behold, what manner of love the Father hath bestowed upon us, that we should be called the sons of God.*

1 John 4:16 *And we have known and believed the love that God hath to us. God is love; and he that dwelleth in love dwelleth in God, and God in him.*

The bottom line is this: Do things unto the Lord. Don't do things so that others will validate and accept and approve of you.

Do what you do because it is what God wants you to do. Fortunately, there's only one person that we need to seek the approval of and that is GOD. Regardless of what other people say or do, God will never leave you nor forsake you even if He does not agree with what you do or say.

Hebrews 13:5 *Let your conversation be without covetousness; and be content with such things as ye have: for He hath said, I will never leave thee, nor forsake thee.*

God loves us all, all of the time, no matter what. He loves us unconditionally. He will never leave or forsake us. Jesus said in:

John 8:29, *"...The Father has not left me alone, for I always do those things that please Him."*

The Bible tells us also that obeying God can also bring us favor with people.

Proverbs 16:7 *"When a man's ways please the LORD, He makes even His enemies to be at peace with him."*

So if we are being honest and we are being doers of the word, if we are pleasing the Lord, even our enemies will be at peace with us.

Psalm 37:4 *Delight thyself also in the LORD: and he shall give thee the desires of thine heart.*

God is aware of the desires of your heart, and as our relationship with Him grows, we can hope for the desires of our hearts. The thing we have to remember is this, when we are in an intimate relationship with God, He will give us the desires of our hearts. The desires that are in our hearts, will line up with God and His word.

If our desire is to have healthy and Godly relationships with other people, God can help us with that. We have to learn to examine our motivations. We have to ask ourselves why we do the things that we are doing. We can think that when we are pleasing other people we are being nice. But we may be people pleasers because of what we expect in return.

If you serve someone else, then do it unto the Lord—not to get something back. If you are looking to other people to make you feel okay about yourself, they become your god. We are in idolatry to them and their thoughts and their behaviors.

The truth is that we don't have to look to other people for our self esteem. God will lift you up. We have to look for what God says about us.

James 4:10 *Humble yourselves in the sight of the Lord, and he shall lift you up.*

We have to trust God to lift us up.

John 3:16 *For God so loved the world, that he gave his only Son, that whoever believes in him should not perish but have eternal life.*

God so loved the world—that is you—you are in the world. God loves you. That is awesome, the Creator of the world loves you!

If we are looking for other people to give us our self esteem, we are in idolatry to the person. We have set that person up as a god to us. Who needs people to be our gods, when we have the one true God, the Creator of the universe?

Romans 8:31 *If God be for us, who can be against us?*

You have to begin to understand that setting aside your own needs to make sure that you are pleasing someone else so that they do not reject you, is not being honest. It is a lie. When we are doing things for everyone else and we are denying our own needs, we can become bitter and resentful because we are using all of our energy and time to please other people.

When others don't fulfill our expectations of them, we can become angrier and more resentful. We can begin to carry a grudge in our hearts.

An example of this can be that we do all kinds of things for someone that we are in relationship with, at our own expense. In our own minds we think that we are pleasing this person and so they should like us and treat us with respect and kindness. It is almost as if you can think that you are buying an insurance policy. People think that if they perform for the other person, then when they need something the other person will fulfill their expectations. This is doing things for the wrong reasons.

If the person does or says something that we don't like, I have heard people say, "I have been so nice to them, how can they do this to me? I have done everything for them."

We can think that if we are pleasing the other person that they will always fulfill our expectations of them. That is not the truth and it causes a lot of problems in relationships if we are doing things for the wrong reasons and we are looking to get something from the other person.

We have to be honest with ourselves about why we do things. We have to learn to work out our thoughts and feelings with God. Our goal should be to be honest with God and ourselves and with other people. We have to watch our motives. Are we doing things with the right reasons in mind? We have to ask ourselves this question, "Are my motives Godly?"

I have to ask myself this question all of the time. Why am I doing this? Am I trying to please someone so that they will approve of me? Do I really have the time or the energy to do what they are asking me to do? Or, am I just trying to avoid conflict and make sure that the person will not reject me?

These are important questions to ask yourself.

Remember, we don't have to like or want to do everything that we need to do. There are many things that we have to do because we have responsibilities in our lives. For example, we have to get up early to go to work, or we have to take our children to school or we have to take our cars in to be serviced, or we have to pay our bills and clean our homes. These things have nothing to do with being a people pleaser. We don't have to like everything that we do, but we all have responsibilities that we have to do.

We don't have to love every one of our responsibilities, but we have to do them in the right spirit. We have to do things unto the Lord and drop our expectations of other people.

If we do things for people we should do them as unto the Lord. We do them because we love God who first and always loves us, not because we expect the other person to perform for us.

1 John 4:19 *We love him, because he first loved us.*

Bitterness and Unforgiveness

The next personality issue or spiritual issue that we will talk about is bitterness and un-forgiveness. This is a big issue in any disease, but it is a bigger issue in cancer especially.

Here is an article that links anger and unforgiveness with cancer:

Those who hold onto anger and hurt (without expressing it), tend to have poor health, a weakened immune system and are more prone to chronic illness such as cancer. This is due to a rise in the level of the stress hormone cortisol that suppresses the immune system. Cancer is, in most cases, a state of chronic un-forgiveness; a holding onto anger, hate and resentment. This internal state of chronic stress depletes important adrenaline reserves and breaks the all important oxygen krebs cycle of the body's cells, leading to cancer cell mutation[36]." *(It further details these destructive links to cancer.)*

World Research Links Cancer To Un-forgiveness

1. "Chronic un-forgiveness causes stress. Every time people think of their transgressor, their body responds. Decreasing your un-forgiveness cuts down your health risk. Now, if you can forgive, that can actually strengthen your immune system." [Virginia Commonwealth University]

2. "The program's preliminary work suggests that forgiveness lowered the stress hormone cortisol that in turn affects the immune system, but

only when the patients forgave the ones they blamed." [University of Maryland—Institute of Human Virology]

3. "Forgiveness could boost the immune system by reducing the production of the stress hormone cortisol" [Rockefeller University New York]

4. "When you hold onto the bitterness for years, it stops you from living your life fully. As it turns out, it wears out your immune system and hurts your heart" [Stanford University Center for Research in Disease Prevention]

5. "Those who received forgiveness training showed improvements in the blood flow to their hearts" [University of Wisconsin—Research Dept]

6. Researchers at the University of Michigan's Institute for Social Research found that forgiveness was linked with better self-reported mental and physical health.

7. A new study from Duke University Medical Center demonstrates that those who forgive others experience lower levels of chronic pain and less associated psychological problems like anger and depression than those who have not forgiven.

8. Researchers at Ohio States University found that the highly stressed women had lower levels of natural killer cells than women who reported less stress. "Natural killer cells have an extremely important function with regard to cancer because they are capable of

detecting and killing cancer cells. Psychological interventions, such as forgiveness, have important roles in reducing stress and improving quality of life, but also in extending survival." [Barbara Andersen, Professor of Psychology, Ohio State University]

9. "I have collected 57 extremely well documented so-called cancer miracles. At a certain particular moment in time they decided that the anger and the depression were probably not the best way to go, since they had such little time left. And so they went from that to being loving, caring, no longer angry, no longer depressed, and able to talk to the people they loved. These 57 people had the same pattern. They gave up, totally, their anger, and they gave up, totally, their depression, by specifically a decision to do so. And at that point the tumors started to shrink." [Yale Medical School—Dr. Bernie Seigel, Clinical Professor of Surgery]

10. "When I suggest emotional healing to people with cancer, they always misunderstand me. They hear it as emotional support. They think I either just want to comfort them, or show them how to have a more positive attitude. They don't get that something like forgiveness might be the key to their getting well. I see their eyes glaze over when I go on to say that emotional toxicity is most likely the cause of their cancer, and that forgiveness, if used with appropriate treatments and lifestyle changes that address the physical, is a 'first-line' primary treatment. Their inability to hear this as a strategy for survival, is a measure of how brainwashed we all are into thinking that treatment for cancer

must always be harsh, drastic and violent. With our War-on-Cancer mind-set, it's hard to imagine that something so seemingly soft and gentle as forgiveness could be the answer to our problem." [Colin Tipping, Director, Institute of Radical Forgiveness]

When we look at this information that these articles show us, it is so clear that bitterness and un-forgiveness is a real problem. It definitely can affect our health.

When someone has cancer, this spirit of bitterness seems to drive the person. It comes out of self centered thinking and self focused behaviors. These people are very stuck in what they think should happen, what others should say, and what others should do and what others should think. They have expectations of others and when these expectations are not fulfilled they become angry. They generally just simmer inside.

They may not say anything to the person that has done something that they did not like, but they are really angry and offended. They can seem to be passive aggressive in their demonstration of their anger. For example, they will tell you that they will meet you at 4:00 and come at 5:00 or they will retaliate by talking about you or not answering your phone calls.

They can gossip about you, give you the silent treatment, say something mean, put you down in conversation, be sarcastic or cold, etc. They do not deal with the offense head on but they want to retaliate, they do it in an underground way, never really dealing with the truth.

It is almost as if they just don't have the ability to deal with things in a constructive and Godly way. The truth is that they don't have the skills to deal with their issues in a Godly way. They did not see healthy behavior and relationship skills in their family of origin.

These people have had problems in childhood but they have not tried to deal with them. They pretty much live a lie that all is well and they don't touch their pain. They are programmed to get irritated, angry, hold grudges and to retaliate. Remember this word "programmed." Think of programming a computer. We program the computer to do things in a particular way, and that is what the computer will do. Our minds are similar. We are creatures of habit and we can be programmed to do things that line up with Satan and his kingdom.

People can be just unaware of this. They are generally unaware that there is another way to behave. We know that in the Bible, God tells us a lot about forgiving others. Here are just a few scriptures:

Matthew 6:14-15 *For if you forgive others their trespasses, your heavenly Father will also forgive you, but if you do not forgive others their trespasses, neither will your Father forgive your trespasses.*

Matthew 18:21-22 *Then Peter came up and said to him, "Lord, how often will my brother sin against me, and I forgive him? As many as seven times?" Jesus said to him, "I do not say to you seven times, but seventy times seven.*

Luke 23:34 *And Jesus said, "Father, forgive them, for they know not what they do." And they cast lots to divide his garments.*

Colossians 3:12-13 *Put on then, as God's chosen ones, holy and beloved, compassionate hearts, kindness, humility, meekness, and patience, bearing with one another and, if one has a complaint against another, forgiving each other; as the Lord has forgiven you, so you also must forgive.*

1 John 1:9 *If we confess our sins, he is faithful and just to forgive us our sins and to cleanse us from all unrighteousness.*

God wants us to forgive others. We can expect to suffer if we do not. It is also important to remember that it is okay to be angry and it is okay to express our feelings and thoughts about issues in our lives that hurt us. We have to be aware of not sinning when we do have these issues to work out.

The last thing that I want to emphasize is that it is not okay to have people thinking that it is wrong to be angry. It is okay to be angry. It is what you do with your anger that will make all of the difference in your life and in relationships with others as well.

When I meet someone who has a chronic health problem, I know that in some way they are harboring un-forgiveness. Now, I want to make something clear here and that is that sometimes people don't understand forgiveness. They think that it means that you should never be angry at anyone. They think that they can never talk about their feelings or their hurts.

This is not true.

We have discussed the scripture, "be angry and sin not," It is not a sin to be angry. The problems come when we do not deal with our anger in a Godly way.

Here are two scriptures that tell us what to do when we have hurts in our hearts:

James 5:16 *Confess your faults one to another, and pray one for another, that ye may be healed.*

Matthew 5:4 *Blessed are they that mourn: for they shall be comforted.*

These two scriptures alone tell us what to do. We find someone whom we can trust and we confess our faults one to another. It is okay to mourn and tell someone all about our hurts and trials and pains. It is okay to cry or to express our feelings one to another.

We must take our hurts and concerns to God.

Philippians 4:6 *Be careful for nothing; but in everything by prayer and supplication with thanksgiving let your requests be made known unto God.*

We are to tell God about everything, and that includes telling Him all about all of our feelings and our thoughts. In Psalm 69 where David is telling God all about his problems and his distresses and trials and tribulations. You can read this entire Psalm and see exactly what David is telling his Father God, in heaven. Starting in verse 22, David is telling God how he feels about his enemies:

²²Let their table become a snare before them: and that which should have been for their welfare, let it become a trap. ²³Let their eyes be darkened, that they see not; and make their loins continually to shake. ²⁴Pour out thine indignation upon them, and let thy wrathful anger take hold of them. ²⁵Let their habitation be desolate; and let none dwell in their tents. ²⁶For they persecute him whom thou hast smitten; and they talk to the grief of those whom thou hast wounded. ²⁷Add iniquity unto their iniquity: and let them not come into thy righteousness. ²⁸Let them be blotted out of the book of the living, and not be written with the righteous.

When we read about David, there is not a question about how he is feeling about his enemies. He is mad and he is expressing his anger and he is actually cursing them.

Is David wrong to do this or to say this? NO. He is just telling God his feelings. He is confessing his thoughts one to another. He is mourning and is sharing his broken heart. He is confessing, he is mourning. He is talking to God. He is working out his issues with God. In Psalm 69 starting in verse 29 David begins to talk to God about how he is going to resolve these feelings:

²⁹But I am poor and sorrowful: let thy salvation, O God, set me up on high. ³⁰I will praise the name of God with a song, and will magnify him with thanksgiving. ³¹This also shall please the LORD better than an ox or bullock that hath horns and hoofs. ³²The humble shall see this, and be glad: and your heart shall live that seek God. ³³For the LORD heareth the poor, and despiseth not his prisoners. ³⁴Let the heaven and earth praise him, the seas, and everything that moveth therein. ³⁵For God will save Zion, and will build the cities of Judah: that they may dwell there, and have it in possession. ³⁶The seed also of his servants shall inherit it: and they that love his name shall dwell therein.

David is now praising God. He gave all his urgent concerns and powerful emotions to God, giving the entire situation to God. He is trusting his Father in heaven.

My point is this. We can be angry, we can mourn and we can confess our sins to someone else or to God, but in the end we have to know that God is going to take care of the situation for us. It is our job to have a heart to forgive and let God take over.

The right of vengeance belongs to the Lord.

Romans 12:9 *Dearly beloved, avenge not yourselves, but rather give place unto wrath: for it is written, Vengeance is mine; I will repay, saith the Lord.*

We have to let God deal with other people, it is our job to learn how to forgive and give the problem to God.

When I meet someone who has a chronic health problem, the first thing that I look for is un-forgiveness.

When someone is hurt or has a problem, sometimes people want to be all religious and hyper-spiritual and self righteous. We can try to confess our hurts to someone and they might tell us that we are into bitterness and un-forgiveness and they can tell us to repent for being bitter.

But if the person has not dealt with their feelings and they have just denied or suppressed or repressed their anger and no amount of repenting will help them. They are still harboring un-forgiveness in their hearts.

If the person does not have experience with dealing with their hurts and anger in Godly ways, they can repent, but they may still have the same patterns of behavior that will come out when something happens that makes them angry. They still may have a broken heart because of the hurts that they have had.

The truth is that we can't repent for un-forgiveness and bitterness if we don't even acknowledge our own thoughts and feelings and work out our issues with God in a Godly way. We have to learn new ways of thinking and behaving.

Forgiving someone does not mean that we condone what they did. It does not mean that what they did didn't hurt and affect us. It just means that we are going to let the issue go. We are going to go on with our lives and let God handle the issue.

One thing that I always say about un-forgiveness is that it is like shooting yourself in the foot and waiting for the other person to limp. Holding onto un-forgiveness is just not good for your health. When people do not deal with the un-forgiveness in their heart they can simmer inside of their heart. The un-forgiveness turns into resentment and then the anger is still remaining inside of their heart. They can simmer and simmer. They can be harboring rage.

Sometimes people don't forgive and move on ... they just move on with their un-forgiveness. They move on without ever really dealing with their issues and they keep their inability to have healthy relationships.

So, when we are angry and we don't face our feelings and work them out with God, we can let our anger and hurt simmer inside of our hearts and we can be setting ourselves up for sickness and disease.

Bitterness and un-forgiveness is a dangerous thing. It can lead to resentment, wrath, grudges, violence and eventually murder. It lets the principality of bitterness have a place in our lives.

Every time I minister to someone who has cancer they have problems dealing with anger. They deny, suppress, repress or ignore their anger and rage. No matter how they handle their anger, the common denominator is that they don't know how to deal with their hurts and their anger. They don't know how to come to peace with their anger and bitterness.

Whether they are in denial or they are raging, they are still stuck on thinking that things have to go their way. They still feel entitled to have things go their way and they are not flexible enough to let things go. They are still not dealing with things in a Godly way.

I remember when I began to understand this personality pattern of being angry and simmering, I remembered an event that stands out in my mind.

I once asked a secretary to look up a telephone number. She did look up the number for me, and she did it with a smile (which was the lie) and yet she really did not want to do it at all. I could see the resentment and irritation on her face and I could hear it in her voice. She had a spirit of bitterness rise up and she was truly irritated and angry inside, she felt put upon. She really did not want to look up the number—which was her job—and yet, she did it, but she continued to simmer inside.

This was her job and she knew that she was supposed to look up the number, but she really did not want to do it. The problem was not that she was irritated or angry; it was that she did not do anything about the simmering. It just hung around.

She moved on with the anger still in her heart. I could see it in her face and her tone of voice after she gave me the number. I irritated her with my request. Irritation leads to anger.

What we should do is to try to understand and reason why you become irritated, annoyed or angry in the first place so that you can deal with these issues with God. We have to face the truth about what we think and feel and work out our issues with God and His word guiding us.

An important piece of information that I have learned is that irritation actually leads to anger. There is a thin line of difference between irritation and anger. Irritation is exasperation and it leads us right into anger. It can be the start of that simmering of anger and irritation and annoyance that can leave you stressed and hassled. It can lead you to experience personality conflicts; it can lead to having you feel undervalued and powerless. It can leave you feeling annoyed and that the other person crossed your boundaries and yet you don't think that you can do anything about it.

The problem that we recognize here in the experience with the secretary is that the person did not work out their feelings with God. She was not in peace about what she was doing.

It is not the fact that you have a feeling or a thought that is the problem; it is how you deal with that feeling or thought that makes all the difference. Your thought or feeling is not sin, unless you let it hang around and you get into agreement with it.

We can be angry and we can be irritated, but we have to work out our feelings with God and come to a place of peace. We have to be flexible and have patience and having the other fruits of the Spirit become our nature.

The secretary was irritated and angry, but she did not work out her issue with God. She had a perpetual irritation about her. I just knew that when I asked her to do something that it would irritate her. Remember this scripture: (I know that I refer to it a lot, but God put it in the Bible so that we would know His heart.)

Ephesians 4:26 *Be ye angry, and sin not: let not the sun go down upon your wrath.*

We can look at this scripture and we can substitute other feelings for the anger. We can say, "Be irritated and sin not," but don't let too much time go by before working this situation and thoughts and feelings out with God.

We can say, "Be aggravated and sin not" but don't let too much time go by before you work out this situation with God.

When the scripture says do not let the sun go down on your wrath it does not mean that we can't be angry when the sun goes down. It is really telling us to work out our issues with God as soon as we can. Don't let your anger hang out and slip into wrath and hatred and revenge and violence and eventually murder. We are human beings. We are created in God's image, and that includes our God-given capacity to have feelings.

By the way, we can think that anger and wrath have the same definition, but the Bible Dictionary defines anger in this way:

Anger definition: The emotion of instant displeasure on account of something evil that presents itself to our view. In itself it is an original susceptibility of our nature, just as love is, and is not necessarily sinful. It may, however, become sinful when causeless, or excessive, or protracted (Matthew 5:22; Ephesians 4:26; Colossians 3:8). As ascribed to God, it merely denotes His displeasure with sin and with sinners (Psalm 7:11).

Wrath is defined in this way: Wrath applies especially to anger that seeks vengeance or punishment.

So if we allow anger to hang around we can let Satan influence us into becoming resentful and eventually we may want to retaliate or get revenge.

The bottom line is that we should not allow our thoughts and feelings to hang out in our minds without working everything out with God. What is an example of working this situation out with God?

Well, let's say that the secretary did get irritated and angry and she resented having to look up the number for me, she could have said to God, "God, I repent for holding onto my anger. I know that this is my job. But I was stressed out and had a lot to do and I was trying to get everything done. But Father, I know that I can depend on you to help me. I know that I can only do my best. I am going to take my peace and I release this anger and resentment to You. I repent for allowing fear to enter my heart and for trying to be perfect. I release this person who asked me for the number and I ask You to bless them. I know that my joy and peace comes from You Lord and not from my performance."

Then she might have looked to Satan and his kingdom and said, "I know that you want me to get angry and stay angry and irritated and annoyed for ungodly reasons. I know that you want me to hold a grudge, but I am choosing not to do that. I cast you out of my life. Stop talking to me."

Instead of doing this and working out their issues with God, people with this personality trait let the devil influence them and their angers and irritations simmer beneath the surface. Instead of doing things unto the Lord and taking their peace about the situation, they might do something passive aggressive like talk about you or give you the wrong number or ignore you or give you the silent treatment. Their tone of voice and their facial expressions tell the whole story about how angry and irritated they really are. They never really are admitting to themselves that they did not want to do the thing and that they are down-right angry and irritated.

A little side note here when this happened to me, I had a choice to make. I could have taken the secretary's behavior personally or I could have realized that her behavior was about her and her thoughts and feelings and it was not about me.

I chose to know that her behavior was about her and I let the situation go. I thanked her for helping me and I left her with her issues and I did not compound her problem by getting angry or nasty with her.

If you have something that happens to you and you are sad and hurt and you are angry, remember God's word in these scriptures:

Matthew 5:4 *Blessed are they that mourn: for they shall be comforted.*

James 5:16 *Confess your faults one to another, and pray one for another, that ye may be healed.*

God expects us to mourn and to be sad and to be angry. He expects us to cry out to Him and tell Him our problems. God knows that it is healthy for us to tell Him and ourselves the truth about how we think and feel. He expects us to take some time and express our thoughts and feelings to other people.

Our job as family, friends or ministers is to listen with compassion and love and empathy. We should validate the person's feelings and love them. Let them know that you understand how they feel, and point them to God for their solution about how to handle the situation.

Sometimes when people are angry or sad or hurt, they can say things that they don't mean. Give the person a chance to confess their thoughts and feelings. We don't want to judge them and criticize them and pile more guilt and shame on them.

The important thing to remember is that we should always lead them into doing the Godly thing with the situation with which they are dealing.

Another example would be that you might mistakenly say something wrong to a person that hurts their feelings. Let's say that they will not tell you about it, but they will simmer about it. They never deal with the problem it just stays that way in their thinking. They may retaliate by saying something mean in a conversation or by gossiping about you or by being sarcastic to you.

They may also begin to change their behavior towards you. You might notice that they do not seem the same towards you. They will not tell you what is wrong, but you will know something is wrong because of their attitude.

Another example occurred where I ministered to a woman who had cancer and she admitted that she never really told her husband what she liked or disliked. Out of obligation and performance she behaved in the ways that she thought that she was expected to, but beneath the surface she resented him and was angry. She never really tried working out these thoughts or feelings. She just kind of kept everything inside and she was irritated and annoyed most of the time.

Another example is that I prayed for a woman who had breast cancer. She and her three daughters were in the kitchen cooking, and when I walked in you could cut the "discomfort" with a knife. The mother was irritated because she wanted things done her way and the girls were not meeting her expectations.

You could see the irritation on her face and in the way that she was reacting to the girls. All of this was underground and no one was really admitting it or was working out their irritation or anger or letting go of their expectations, disappointments or anger.

All four women were holding in their irritation and anger and no one was saying anything. But you could see the irritation on their faces. You could discern the spirits having a field day. These women were in denial.

Another example shows what can happen when someone holds unto un-forgiveness and irritation. I was ministering to someone who had cancer.

As I ministered to them they said that they had no problems and they did not know why they had cancer. As I spoke with the person, I discerned a spirit of irritation with every question that I asked and every answer that I got. After a while, I realized that this person was just downright irritated. This irritation was part pattern for how they interacted with other people.

Finally, I asked, "Are you irritated with me? Are you annoyed by my questions?" The person's first response was NO. It took awhile and some careful explanations mixed with compassion and love, but the person began to see that they were irritated. They really did not realize that they spoke with irritation in their voice almost all of the time.

This is denial. Remember the acronym: I don't even "no" that I am lying.

Remember that if you are irritated all of the time, your thoughts will cause secretions of chemicals into your body, and this can cause an environment that is conducive to disease. God did not create us to be irritated all of the time and so our bodies will show the consequences or even the curse of that feeling of irritation.

Another example of being angry or irritated and holding onto the anger is a situation that happened to me. Someone wanted me to come to their home. They had a specific time frame that they wanted me to conform to and when I could not conform to their time frame the anger that rose up in them was tangible. I felt their irritation and anger. I know that I was not doing what the person wanted me to do. This person did not acknowledge the anger, nor did they say the truth of how they were feeling. They just continued to ignore the anger that sat between us like a pink elephant. The person continued to try and manipulate me to use their time frame. No matter how hard I tried, the person would not admit their annoyance or irritation or anger.

However, it was noticeable and it was tangible to me and another person who was with me. If we don't admit our issues, we are stuck and we can't quit something that we don't recognize and admit. That anger then can become a way of life, and it will just simmer.

Remember – ADMIT IT, QUIT IT and EXCHANGE IT. We have to recognize and admit our issues that don't line up with God and His word. We have to purpose in our hearts to quit our issues that don't line up with God and His word, and we have to exchange our old thoughts and behaviors with new ones that come from God and His word.

We have been looking at cancer and the personality issues or spiritual issues that we can see present in people who have cancer or who have a propensity to have cancer.

Remember, when we talk about people who have these issues in their personality, they don't necessarily have cancer. Just because you have some of these personality issues or spiritual issues in your personality and thoughts and behaviors, it does not mean that you will get cancer. But, it is certainly going to be practicing disease prevention if we can identify and recognize ways that we think and behave which don't line up with God and His word. We are practicing disease prevention if we purpose in our hearts to change our ways so that what we think and do is in agreement with God and His ways.

The word says this: **3 John 1:2** *Beloved, I wish above all things that thou mayest prosper and be in health, even as thy soul prospereth.*

This scripture tells us about how to have our soul prosper. Remember, our soul is where we have our mind, our will and our emotions. It is where we think, reason, believe, decide and feel. It is also where we have our memories and our patterns of behaviors.

So, if we can get our soul into agreement with God and His word, this scripture tells us that we will prosper and be in health. These teachings are not just for people who have cancer, they are for all of us who want to judge ourselves so that we don't have to wait for God to judge us.

1 Corinthians 11:31 *For if we would judge ourselves, we should not be judged.*

When we listen to teachings and we read the word and we wash with the water of the word and we renew our minds, we are shining the light of God's truth on the areas in our lives that do not line up with God and His word. When we recognize that we have areas that do not line up with God and His word we can then **admit** these things, **quit** these things and **exchange** them with thoughts and behaviors that do line up with God and His word.

That is disease prevention!

Bitterness

To review, we have been discussing cancer and the principality of bitterness. We read some studies that indicated that un-forgiveness is a trait that the researchers saw in the people that they studied who had cancer.

We said that sometimes when people get angry they can slip into resentment and then into carting around grudges and un-forgiveness. They can want to retaliate and take revenge against the person that hurt them. They can slip into violence or murder with the tongue, hand or heart.

The thing that I am learning more and more is that people do what they saw others do when they were growing up. People have patterns and programming that they don't even know that they have. We see what our parents and teachers did, and we emulate what they did. We may not want to emulate them and yet we do, and we don't even know that we are doing it.

I have been giving some examples of situations where we can see how bitterness can affect our health. The examples that I was sharing were about people who hold grudges and don't even know it. When you hold a grudge against someone, it means that they said or did something that you did not like and you are still angry with them. You have not forgiven them. You resent them and in your heart, you have something against them. You are holding a grudge or a record of wrongs against them.

We have to remember that sometimes it does take awhile to work through issues in your life. That is the key to changing. We have to be aware of how we are thinking and feeling about the issues in our lives. No matter what happens we have to be working on our issues with God. If we are angry with someone and we are not trying to work through our issues with God, we can be holding onto un-forgiveness and the principality of bitterness can get into our lives.

So if someone does something or says something to us that we don't like, the first thing that we should be aware of doing is to work the situation out with God. Be honest with God and then choose to do the Godly thing in the situation.

Sometimes we need to share our thoughts and emotions with someone whom we trust. Remember:

James 5:16 *Confess your faults one to another, and pray one for another, that ye may be healed.*

Matthew 5:4 *Blessed are they that mourn: for they shall be comforted.*

Blessed are they who mourn means that we are blessed when we express our sorrow because we can be comforted.

THE BOTTOM LINE IS THIS: The Bible is telling us to communicate and tell the truth about how we think and feel.

Passive-Aggressive Behavior

One of the personality issues that we can see in someone who has cancer is that they can be passive-aggressive. I have seen this personality trait when I minister to people who have cancer. I see this in other diseases, but I see it almost always in someone who has cancer.

Have you ever talked to someone and you just know that they are angry with you or something is just not right with your relationship? You ask them if something is wrong and they just say, "Oh no, nothing is wrong." They may even put a big smile on their face but yet you just know that something is very wrong

You know by the tone of their voice or their facial expressions or how they are treating you with some stand offish attitude. Perhaps they did not call you or they did not pick up the telephone when you called them or they are just giving you the silent treatment.

This person will not tell you what the issue is out of fear or just because they don't have the relationship skills to be honest. They might be holding grudges and they don't feel capable or able or willing to express their thoughts and feelings.

Being passive-aggressive means that instead of confronting a person and a problem directly, up front, I do something negative to hint at the problem in the hope that the other person will get it. I might do something to retaliate against the person to show my anger or to punish them for what they did or said.

It is trying to manipulate, control and retaliate in a roundabout way. The person is not being up front and honest. This can be an example of passive aggressive behavior.

It has been my experience that this is a part of this Type C cancer profile. Remember the Type C profile says that the person doesn't tell the truth about how they feel. It also says that the person is holding onto un-forgiveness. It also says that the person is fabricating their personality so that they will not cause conflict and so that they will be liked.

"Type C" Personality

This is a person that avoids facing and dealing with conflicts and the truth and their true feelings.

Let's review one of the traits that the studies talked about in regard to the Type C PERSONALITY. One of these traits was said to be:

Harboring suppressed toxic emotions (anger, resentment or hostility): These individuals often show an inability to express and resolve deep emotional problems or conflicts and are often unaware of their presence. Read more at Suite101: Personality and cancer: How Personality Impacts Health[37]

The dictionary describes the word "lie" in the following way: v 1. To say something that is not true in a conscious effort to deceive somebody, 2. To give a false impression; n 1. A false statement made deliberately, 2. A false impression created deliberately.

God tells us the bottom line about habitual lying:

Revelation 21:8 *But the fearful, and unbelieving, and the abominable, and murderers, and whoremongers, and sorcerers, and idolaters, and all liars, shall have their part in the lake which burneth with fire and brimstone: which is the second death.*

God says that all liars will have their end in the lake of fire. It is important for us to acknowledge that we have to tell the truth to God and to ourselves and to other people. God is all about telling the truth in our relationships. The truth brings freedom.

John 8:32 *And ye shall know the truth, and the truth shall make you free.*

When we know God's truth, when we understand the truth, when we live in the truth, when we walk in the truth, we are FREE. When we deny the truth or ignore the truth or repress the truth or suppress the truth or even rebel against the truth, we are not FREE and we have opened the door of our lives to the devil and to disease.

People who are passive-aggressive seem to be okay and also to be agreeing with you. They seem to be okay with what you are saying and with what you are asking them to do. They may even seem enthusiastic about what you are saying. But in the end they just don't perform a requested action on time or in a useful way, and they may even work against it. They are just not telling the truth about what is really in their heart.

The problem is that the person can be hostile, irritated, annoyed, angry and/or resentful. Yet they may not know that they are harboring any of this and they may not know exactly why, either.

In some cases, people that are unable to recognize or express their annoyance often don't feel entitled to it; they have learned to let the "little things" pass without taking the time to find out why they are so angry about them. They carry their hurts and irritations and annoyances with them. Because they have low self-esteem, they don't want to do anything to offend someone, so their anger remains. They are simmering inside.

What happens is that the person doesn't show outward anger nor do they appear malicious. At first glance, their behavior appears to be unassuming, gracious and they appear to be really nice.

The problem is that when you are dealing with a passive aggressive person, you can end up feeling frustrated, offended, guilty or confused or just defiled or disliked. When you speak with the person you can think that something is wrong, yet you are not quite sure what it was that was wrong. They will not tell you or be honest with you. In other words, they use nonverbal behavior to express anger or resentment that they can't or won't express verbally.

An example could be showing up very late to a meeting that they didn't really want to attend and then making up excuses for their lateness. They don't want to say that they were late because they are angry and they did not want to attend the meeting, so they show their anger by being late. This is passive-aggressive behavior. It is working out your anger by doing something to retaliate, irritate or annoy or hurt the other person.

Below lists signs and symptoms of passive-aggressive behavior:

- Resentment and opposition to the demands of others that is not stated or dealt with
- Complaining about feeling under-appreciated or cheated

- Procrastination
- Stubbornness
- Inefficiency
- Purposeful memory lapses
- Sullenness
- Irritability
- Cynical attitude
- Rebellion

What leads to passive-aggressive behavior?

Quora[38] offers these insights:

It is thought that a pattern of unassertive and passive behavior is **learned in childhood** as a coping strategy. It is most likely a response to parents who exercised complete control and did not let their child express themselves. To cope, a child will adopt a passive-aggressive behavior pattern.

If, for example, a child openly disagrees with their parent(s) and they are punished for doing so; the child would learn to substitute passive resistance for active resistance. Given a consistent pattern of punishment or rejection when asserting oneself, an individual can learn to become highly adept at passively rebelling."

The person's passive aggressive behaviors can start in the person's childhood where it was unsafe to be direct or, worse, the child was punished or shamed if they were direct and outspoken so they learned to manipulate others to survive. They learned to fabricate and to deny their feelings. Sometimes this behavioral style was simply modeled by a parent and adopted as the family dynamic. It is a familiar spirit and a strong hold in the family.

One definition of being passive-aggressive[39]: Passive-Aggression is a psychological mechanism for handling hostility or anger in an underhanded or devious way that is hard for others to prove. Sometimes the passive-aggressive is aware of what he or she is doing, and other times not."

Passive aggression, as defined in The Angry Smile: The Psychology of Passive Aggressive Behavior in Families, Schools, and Workplaces, 2nd edition, is a deliberate and masked way of expressing covert feelings of anger. Couched in backhanded compliments, insulting gifts, hostile sticky notes, and behind angry smiles, passive aggression involves a variety of behaviors (hence, the overuse of the term) designed to get back at another person without the passive aggressor having to own up to or articulate their true feelings. Passive aggression is motivated by a person's **fear** of expressing anger directly."

People can have a fear of telling the truth about how they really feel or think because they are afraid of conflict. They are afraid of rejection and they can think that if they tell the truth , things will be worse for them than if they lie and fabricate. Some common examples of passive-aggressive behavior are:

- When conversing with someone who is angry at you, they leave out important information which gives you the wrong impression of the true situation.

- Communicating hostility by using humor or sarcasm or jokes made at your expense.
- Talking behind the back of someone in a derogatory or harmful way- gossiping.
- Exaggerating the faults of someone you are in relationship with (behind his or her back) to other people while maintaining "sweetness" toward the person.
- Playing dumb or inadequate to frustrate someone or to gain advantage or control.
- Having endless excuses, justifications, and reasons why things did not go well, it is never your fault.
- Being angry with someone and yet you just make believe nothing is wrong.
- If you don't really like what someone is doing or saying but you never say anything, and you give the person the silent treatment or a dirty look.
- You are angry with what someone said or did, and you don't tell them. However, you are secretly happy when something bad happens to them.
- They say that they forgot to do something that you asked them to do because they did not want to tell the truth that they did not want to do what you asked them to do.
- They can be having a constant negative attitude.
- Being critical and judgmental.
- They can seem to voice exaggerated and persistent complaints of personal misfortune. This is the me, me and the woe is me attitude.
- They are entertaining self-pity.
- They can seem irritable, defensive and resentful.

- They can seem to lack self confidence and self esteem.
- They can blame their own unhappiness on others.
- They blame other people for their lack of time.
- They blame other people for their problems. They don't take responsibility for their own problems.
- They can act sullen or uncommunicative.
- They are not aware that these things are part of their behavior pattern, and it seems normal to them.

When people are passive-aggressive they are angry, they can be holding grudges, or they act as if they are a victim. They just don't like what you are saying and doing and yet they don't choose to be honest and or they don't have the skills to be honest and open and share how they are really feeling with you. They are just acting out in ways that make it difficult or confusing to have a relationship with them. They can seem to "punish" those around them in non-confrontational ways. For example, instead of just saying, "I do not want to do what you are asking me to do," they might show up an hour late and sulk about something they are missing in order to help you. They frequently play the "martyr" and "victim" in their relationships.

Another example can be that a man can be upset with his wife's weight gain, and he "affectionately" calls her "pork chop" in public in a way that appears playful on the surface. In reality, this hurts her.

Another example can be that your family member may tell you that they will attend your friend's party, but he or she does not start getting ready to go on time and because of that you are very late. He or she knows this upsets you but either feigns an apology or becomes defensive.

Another example can be a family member is asked to go to the grocery store but returns with only half of the items on the list. He or she may buy items that, that they know you don't want to buy, such as their favorite unhealthy food items, but not the bran cereal you requested. If asked to wash your car, they may deliberately scratch it. The bottom line of this behavior is that they want you to perform the task yourself rather than ask them to do it.

Another example can be that the person with passive-aggressive behavior allows you to make a bad decision, and, when ramifications occur for you, he or she seems pleased and lets you know that they were aware you were making a mistake. For example, you are driving with this person and you take the wrong exit off the interstate and drive 10 miles before you realize you are in the wrong place. As you turn around, he or she lets you know that they knew you were going the wrong way all along.

When we are dealing with someone who has a behavior pattern of being passive-aggressive, the hardest part of the relationship is figuring out how the person really feels. You may leave an interaction with them feeling confused, angry or upset, but you are not quite sure why you feel that way. It can be a confusing relationship because you know that there is something that they are just not saying to you.

Bottom line is the person is angry and they won't tell the truth or they won't admit that they are angry. They don't give you the chance to work things out with them. They just don't have the relationship skills to work out conflicts with other people.

The person's actions can frustrate you and confuse you. They can work hard at retaliating against you in passive ways. Then what happens is that they are actually getting you to act out their angry feelings—to explode and appear crazy— while the passive aggressive person sits back and watches the emotional outburst with satisfaction, total control, and always with their own poise intact.

They have not done anything according to them, and you are the one who is in the wrong. What can happen is that the passive-aggressive person is angry and holding a grudge against you. They are doing things that hurt and confuse you and yet they won't admit to it. This is their way of working out their anger and retaliating or punishing you. This can make you feel crazy and you don't really have a way of working out the situation when the person refuses to deal with the situation in an honest way. So, you eventually get angry and then you are the one to blame for the problems in the relationship.

I want to give some other examples of holding onto a grudge and being passive aggressive and what it looks like. Here is a story that I read: (Author Unknown)

"Cash, check or charge?" I asked, after folding the items the woman wished to purchase. As she fumbled for her wallet, I noticed a remote control for a television set in her purse. "So, do you always carry your TV remote?" I asked. "No," she replied, "but my husband refused to go shopping with me and I figured this was the most evil thing I could do to him legally."

Another example of this is an experience that happened to me. I am going to describe it because it fits the profile, and this person who the story is about has had cancer four times in four different ways in her body.

This happened years ago, but I never forgot it because it so profoundly fits the profile of the kind of thing that I see when people have passive aggressive behavior.

Anyway, I was going on a trip with this person. We were planning to stay at the person's family member's house when we got to our destination. We discussed the trip a lot before we went. We had planned everything that we could, especially sleeping arrangements.

We knew that at our destination there were two places to sleep in the house. One was a small office with a single mattress on the floor. It was not great accommodations, but it was private and it was a place to sleep. The other place to sleep was a basement family room with a pull-out sofa. The basement room was a family room that had another bedroom that my friend's 18 year old nephew was living in. It had a door that opened out into the room where the sofa was where one of us would sleep. The basement also had a washer and dryer and a cat litter box where the cats came all day and night. The young man's bedroom opened up into the room where the sofa was and he could and did come out of his room to go to the bathroom during the night and early in the morning.

Before we went on the trip I said very clearly that I did not want to stay in the basement, for various reasons. The main being that it was not comfortable for me to be sleeping where her nephew could walk in and out. She agreed to this. When we got to our destination she changed her mind and she wanted me to sleep in the basement. I reiterated our agreement and said that I just could not sleep down there for the many reasons we had discussed.

She was irritated. Her irritation turned into anger. I did not go along with her plan and she was angry. She wanted to sleep in the small room. For several days she gave me the silent treatment, she put me down in conversations and she gossiped about me. She was sarcastic. I tried to discuss the issue, but she could not and would not admit that she was angry. She would smile and say nothing was wrong.

The point is that she lied to me and held bitterness in her heart because she did not get what she truly wanted. She resented me. Then— most importantly—she retaliated and would not admit anything was wrong when I asked her. I tried to talk to her and bring the issue out into the open, but she would not discuss the issue. She would not even admit that something was wrong or that she was angry.

This made me very uncomfortable and it was confusing, to say the least.

This is the thing that I think is so noticeable in the personality and behavior of people who have this pattern. The pattern is that they don't really explore their feelings and set them right with God. They are not honest. They have the self centered thinking and then bitterness—they wanted things to go their way—and they have no flexibility for anything else.

The irritation or anger or resentment comes and they are in agreement with it and it simmers beneath the surface. They will retaliate (which is passive-aggressive), even if it is just a facial expression. They almost act like a "saint" (like they are giving a perfect performance). They are fabricating and they are suffering in silence. They don't have the relationship skills to discuss the issue and they don't have the flexibility to be able to be okay when they don't get their own way.

The problem is that people do not know how to feel their feelings in the way that God intended for us to feel our feelings. They hide what they feel. They do not know how to deal with feelings and stress in a normal, healthy and Godly way. While they were growing up they saw people denying their feelings, repressing their feelings and suppressing their feelings. They were never asked about what they thought or felt. If they tried to share how they felt, it caused conflict or strife. They were just expected to perform in the way that their parents expected them to, and they really never learned how to discern what they were really thinking or feeling or how to deal with it.

They were taught to avoid conflict. They saw that if they started a conflict then the end result would be that things would not go too well. At the same time, they were taught to be very selfish and self focused. They were not taught how to be flexible and how to take their peace or how to be okay in whatever situation that they found themselves to be in.

They were taught how to think and behave by watching the adults in their lives. They emulated their parents. They emulated their teachers and their peers. They learned how to lie. They learned how to fabricate and perform.

On the outside they smile but on the inside they are simmering. They are in fear, or they are angry, disappointed, irritated, or annoyed, and generally very self-focused. They are confused and they feel badly and don't even know why.

They can't seem to get their minds off of themselves and what they want or what they think that others should say or do. They can't drop their expectations of others or what they wanted to happen in the situation that did not happen.

I have seen people who get sick every time someone does something that they do not like. They don't see their part in the pattern. An example that I can give is a person who seems to be okay and not in any pain, then someone does something that they do not like and in a short period of time—from immediately to 24 or 48 hours—they get pain in their body.

They have no idea why they are in pain. What actually can happen is that the person is so unaware of their anger and it simmers in their body and they somaticize the anger as pain.

What this means is that their brain feels the emotional pain in their body. Their body is showing the emotional pain that they did not deal with in their minds.

Your body will speak what is in your mind.

If you try and get them to deal with an issue that is controversial or causes stress or conflict, it is like trying to nail Jell-O to the wall. They just wiggle all over the place and they seem to never really face the issue. They use a lot of techniques to avoid dealing with the truth, they deny the issue, they deny that there is a problem, they blame you for the problem, they tell you that you are too emotional, they tell you that there is no problem, and they refuse to face the issue. Sometimes they even get angry with you for trying to make them face the truth.

What they actually do amounts to abuse. However, they are unaware that they are abusing others with their behavior.

It is abusive when you are in a relationship with someone and you are not allowed to discuss issues honestly and openly and deal with the truth. It is abusive when someone does not allow you to discuss issues with them or communicate with them.

When I learned this I began to see how people can be abusing each other and they do not even know it.

Here are some of the ways that people can avoid facing and dealing with conflicts and the truth and their true feelings. The following were adapted from "The Verbally Abusive Relationship" by Patricia Evans[40]:

- **Withholding Information** and not listening empathetically prevents the proper level of intimacy in the relationship from developing.
- **Countering** contradicts what the other person says; the person refuses to accept that the victim's point of view may be valid.
- **Discounting** the victim's feelings of hurt at the abuse implies that there is something wrong with the victim if he feels that way.
- **Disguising verbal abuse as a joke** again invalidates the victim's perceptions.
- **Blocking and diverting** allows the abuser to avoid discussing things that the victim believes are important.
- **Accusing and blaming** the victim unfairly can make the victim believe that she has caused the abuse.
- **Trivializing** the victim's thoughts, ideas and achievements can make the victim feel worthless.
- **Undermining** of the victim by the abuser erodes the person's self confidence.
- **Every threat** made by the abuser is a form of control. The abuser plays on the victim's deepest fears.

- **Forgetting** promises, agreements or previous discussions prevents the victim from talking to the abuser about his behavior.
- **Denial** is a stronger form of forgetting: the abuser denies that any abuse has ever taken place, invalidating the victim's reality and perceptions.
- **Abusive Anger** allows the abuser to release tension and feel power over his victim but increases the victim's anxiety and feelings of failure.

Another way is that they punish you by not talking to you. They reject you. Somehow they just will not face or deal with the issue. The bottom line is that they don't know how to deal with conflict in a Godly way.

The biggest problem is that they just don't know how to behave. They just don't have the relationship skills that lead to an honest and healthy relationship. They just keep doing the same things over and over again even though these things do not work too well for them.

They have a facade that everything is okay, but the truth is that they have very poor communication and relationship skills.

This is one of the traits that people who have cancer seem to have. They act as if everything is okay—which is the lie—when things are not okay at all.

Our lives are all about relationships. Our lives are about our relationship with God, with ourselves and with other people. When we have problems in any of these areas of our lives, these issues can lead to sickness and disease. TRUTH should always be at the base of all relationships. Without it we have no trust and without trust there is no respect or love.

Our Emotions

Psychotherapist Dr. Lawrence LeShan said, "... Individuals with cancer often show the traits of passivity, despair, and suppression of emotional expression."

This substantiates what we have been discussing. The personality style of suppressing our emotions and not facing what we really think and feel, is a trait that Dr. LeShan saw in his patients that have cancer.

When we don't face the truth about how we are feeling we can be anxious and/or depressed and our bodies can suffer the consequences of our thoughts and behaviors. So what can we do to prevent ourselves from having an environment in our bodies that can lead to cancer?

The first step is to renew our minds with God's word. Wash your mind with the water of the word.

- Be aware of what you are thinking.
- Be aware of what you are feeling.
- Decide to be honest with yourself and with God and with other people.
- Learn how to communicate honestly with God and with yourself and with other people.
- Allow yourself and others to mourn so that you will be comforted.

- Allow yourself and others to confess their faults one to another without judgment and criticism.
- Learn how to say the truth in love to the people with whom we have relationships.

Ephesians 4:15 *But speaking the truth in love.*

It helps someone more if we are honest with them, than if we just hold in all of our feelings and don't tell the truth about how we feel.

As God tells us:

Proverbs 27:5 *Open rebuke is better than secret love.*

And be gracious in our speech with others.

Proverbs 15:1 *A soft answer turneth away wrath: but grievous words stir up anger.*

Our goal is to say the truth to people with the love of the Lord.

Remember to let people express their feelings to you. We don't want to accuse them and we don't want to judge them. Our goal is to listen to them and love them and lead them to God and His ways, in love.

I have heard people say that if we don't have something nice to say to someone, we should not say anything at all. This is teaching us to lie and it is not at all what the Bible says.

The Bible says that we should confess our faults one to another and that we should say the truth in love. If we have a problem with our brother or sister we should go to them and communicate with them. We have to learn to communicate with other people in love and with empathy and compassion and with respect.

The truth is that we have to learn how to have the fruits of the Spirit as our nature. Out of our relationship and fellowship with God, our goal is to develop the fruits of the Spirit as our own nature.

Galatians 5:22-23 *But the fruit of the Spirit is love, joy, peace, longsuffering, gentleness, goodness, faith, meekness, temperance.*

These nine fruits are important fruits or qualities that are coming directly from God Himself. Our goal is to work with God so that all nine of these fruits are part of our nature and personality.

God wants all of us to have a true and intimate relationship with Him. He wants us to begin a process of change and sanctification with Him. Our goal is to recognize our old thoughts and behaviors and work with God to begin the process where these changes can be molding, shaping, and transforming us into the image of His Son Jesus Christ. The way that we can work with God to be transformed or changed is by the renewing of our minds. He wants to put right and Godly thinking into our thought processes.

We have to learn to follow God and His word and be honest with Him and with ourselves and with other people. We have to learn to be honest and know what we are really thinking and feeling.

Telling the Truth

When we talked about the articles and studies and the issues that the medical community found in the Type C personality, we saw that the researchers said that these were some of the issues that they saw in a person who could have a propensity to develop cancer. The person can be: "a feeling denier, avoider, suppressor, or repressor, stoic or fabricate their personality. He or she can have a calm, outwardly rational, and unemotional demeanor, but also a tendency to conform to the wishes of others, a lack of assertiveness, and an inclination toward feelings of helplessness or hopelessness."

Most everything that we see in this list relates to not telling the truth to ourselves or to God or to other people.

Let's look at this scripture:

Galatians 1:10 *For do I now persuade men, or God? or do I seek to please men? for if I yet pleased men, I should not be the servant of Christ.*

What this is saying is: Am I now trying to win the approval of men or of God? If I am trying to please men, then I am not a servant of Christ.

We want to be servants of God and not men. Our goal is to follow God and work with Him so that we can be transformed and changed into the image of Jesus.

—— CHAPTER FOUR ——

Satan's Favorite Weapons

The next issues that I would like to discuss about are some of Satan's favorite weapons. They are: selfishness, envy, jealousy, covetousness, lust and the evil eye.

These characteristics or personality patterns can be in our personalities that lead to sickness and disease.

Selfishness

To begin this part of our discussion, I begin with selfishness and related issues. Some of these characteristics are: pride, envy, jealousy, covetousness, comparison, the evil eye and a sense of entitlement.

Whew, this may seem as if it is a lot to look at, but I see this as a mix of problems. It is a way of thinking. It is a way of being programmed to think. I see this as being a very big problem in the people to who I minister that have this disease process. I don't only see it in cancer, but in other diseases as well. These issues are more common than we may think.

Let me give you some examples from scripture of people being selfish:

Genesis 4:9 *And the LORD said unto Cain, Where is Abel thy brother? And he said, I know not: Am I my brother's keeper?*

Cain could care less where his brother was. He was selfish. Another example is:

Mark 10:35-37 *And James and John, the sons of Zebedee, come unto him, saying, Master, we would that thou shouldest do for us whatsoever we shall desire. And he said unto them, What would ye that I should do for you? They said unto him, Grant unto us that we may sit, one on thy right hand, and the other on thy left hand, in thy glory.*

James and John were thinking of their own selfish ambition. Here is another example:

Luke 10:29-32 *But he, willing to justify himself, said unto Jesus, And who is my neighbour? And Jesus answering said, A certain man went down from Jerusalem to Jericho, and fell among thieves, which stripped him of his raiment, and wounded him, and departed, leaving him half dead. And by chance there came down a certain priest that way: and when he saw him, he passed by on the other side. And likewise a Levite, when he was at the place, came and looked on him, and passed by on the other side.*

The priest and the Levite just walked past the person that obviously needed help. That is selfishness.

No one is immune to selfishness. These examples are just a few of many that we can find in the Bible. We see it in Cain's cold-blooded words concerning Abel, we see selfishness in James and John seeking high position in the Kingdom, and we see it when we see the priest and the Levite passing by the wounded man.

Satan's nature is self-centered, and his goal is to influence people to be just like him. Selfishness is all around us. We all have it in different degrees. The Bible tells us all about selfishness in the last days:

> **2 Timothy 3:1-5** *¹This know also, that in the last days perilous times shall come. ²For men shall be lovers of their own selves, covetous, boasters, proud, blasphemers, disobedient to parents, unthankful, unholy, ³Without natural affection, trucebreakers, false accusers, incontinent, fierce, despisers of those that are good, ⁴Traitors, heady, high-minded, lovers of pleasures more than lovers of God; Having a form of godliness, but denying the power thereof: from such turn away.*

Here is another scripture that speaks to this very issue of selfishness:

> **Philippians 2:21** *For all seek their own, not the things which are Jesus Christ's.*

This tells us a lot about what is happening and what is going to happen and how people will act out their selfishness.

I suggest that you take each of these works in Timothy and define them using your Bible dictionary and Bible concordance. This can help us all to take a real good look at ourselves and decide if we do these things or not.

Paul writes that in the last days, selfishness will appear as self-love, self-seeking, and selfish-ambition. Some people will not even consider what they can do for someone else, they are only going to look at what others can do for them. They will look at what more they can get for themselves.

What is selfishness? Selfishness is having too much concern with one's own welfare or interests and too little or no concern for others. We often refer to this type of person as self-centered, self-absorbed, and self-serving. The medical community would label this type of self absorption to be narcissism.

I am going to offer a brief description of what this kind of thinking looks like and then I am going to discuss each issue. I want to expose the devil and how he thinks so that we can recognize these issues in our own lives and decide to quit them and exchange them with thoughts and behaviors that God tells us about in His word. These are issues that have a tendency to hide out and we are not aware that they are in our lives.

Briefly, when we are selfish and self centered, we could say that we are prideful, as well. When we are prideful, we are thinking that we are the most important person in the world. We can be self focused and self centered and we can think that we are entitled to having everything that we want. We can be covetous. We can want everything that everyone else has. We see everything in terms of ourselves. It can be hard for us to be happy for other people who are happy or have what we think that we want, need or are entitled to have. We can have the lust of the flesh and lust of the eyes in our hearts. We can be looking at the things in the world and want them and covet them and lust after them. We may not just covet and lust after things or objects; we can look at other people's relationships and covet them for ourselves. We can be comparing ourselves to other people and we can want what they have. We can be very unhappy because they have what we want, and we don't have it. We can be angry that other people have what we want and we can wish that they did not have what we want. If they have what we want, and we don't have it, we can feel even worse. There is an old saying: Misery loves company. If we can't have it, we don't want others to have it. The person can be thinking, "If I am not going to get what I want, I don't want you to have it either."

This is a whole mix of ways of thinking that definitely do not line up with God and His word. It can be confusing, so let's look at each individual issue and then put it together so we can see what this really looks like.

Let's start by looking at selfishness: a selfish self-focus is what starts this whole thing off. Here is a definition of selfishness: Selfishness is defined by the dictionary as a focus on one's own pleasure or well-being without regard for others.

Satan wants to influence us to be selfish, self centered and self focused. This can come along with self-pity and a sense of entitlement. This is when people think that they are entitled to have things go their way. If things do not go their own way, they are really irritated, disappointed and angry.

They become hopeless because they have not gotten what they wanted and they can't seem to be flexible and change their mind about what they want. They don't see how they can go on without having things be the way that they want them to be.

Sometimes, people want what they want and if they don't get what they want, they become really disappointed. It is not a problem to be disappointed. The problem arises when we don't deal with the disappointment with God as soon as we can.

People also in our day have a growing sense of entitlement. There's an ever-increasing number of children growing up with a selfish sense of Entitlement, children refusing to grow up, thinking the world owes them what they desire.

Entitlement

Entitlement or a 'Sense of Entitlement' is an unrealistic, unmerited or inappropriate expectation of favorable living conditions and favorable treatment at the hands of others. A belief that one is entitled to certain benefits.

In clinical psychology and psychiatry an unrealistic, exaggerated, or rigidly held sense of entitlement may be considered a symptom of Narcissistic Personality Disorder.

I am going to define Narcissistic Personality Disorder because remember, the medical and psychological community does a good job defining illnesses and diseases and disorders. They do a great job defining the results of Satan and his kingdom in the lives of men. Remember, God can heal and the medical community can define. Just because the medical community defines a problem and prophecies about it, however, that does not mean that God can't heal the problem. Always remember what God tells us in scripture:

Matthew 19:26 *But Jesus beheld them, and said unto them, With men this is impossible; but with God all things are possible.*

Mark 9:23 *Jesus said unto him, If thou canst believe, all things are possible to him that believeth.*

To continue on here is a brief definition of narcissism: a mental disorder characterized by extreme self-absorption, an exaggerated sense of self-importance, and a need for attention and admiration from others. It is characterized by self-preoccupation, lack of empathy, and unconscious deficits in self-esteem.

Covetousness and Lust

What all of this means is this, we can think that we are entitled to get what we want when we want it. And, if we don't get what we want when we want it, we can get very disappointed and angry and hopeless and jealous. We can be entertaining covetousness, lust of life and lust of the flesh and finally, just lust in general. Lust does not come from God. It come from the world, the flesh, and the devil.

1 John 2:16 *For all that is in the world, the lust of the flesh, and the lust of the eyes, and the pride of life, is not of the Father, but is of the world.*

When we lust after anything, when we are covetous and we think that we just have to have things our way we are opening ourselves up to things that are not from God. They are things of the world and Satan and his kingdom. It is the "it's all about me" complex that gets us into trouble.

When I was doing research about this, I came across another psychological definition of a disorder it was called the "Acquired Self-centered Syndrome (ASS)."

Acquired Self-centered Syndrome (ASS) is not a new "disorder" it's been around ever since Eve bit into the forbidden fruit in the Garden of Eden. Adam followed Eve's lead and also ate of the forbidden fruit.

Eve ate the fruit because, well, she wanted to be like God. Who else do we know that wanted to be like God? Lucifer had a "pride goeth before the fall moment" and he boasted, *"I will ascend above the tops of the clouds; I will make myself like the Most High"* (Isaiah 14:14).

Lucifer, the Prince of Demons, was a guy who wanted to be like God.

With Adam and Eve's rebellion, the personal pronoun "I" or "me" was heard. It's all about me, what I feel, what my needs are, and my desires. It all boils down to this—I, me, my. The ideas are, "It's all about me," and "I am entitled to get whatever

I want." When we are selfish and self focused, somewhere along the line in our lives, we have probably decided that we were entitled to have whatever it is that we want.

You may have decided that people have to say and do what you want them to say and do. You decided that if they don't, then you have the right to be angry. As a matter of fact, you may have decided that you are entitled to be angry. You may have decided that the person who stood in the way of your wants and desires needs to be punished.

In other words, you are entitled to get what you want. If you don't, you get and stay angry and disappointed. You get hopeless and helpless because you don't know how to be flexible and accept things as they are. You don't know how to change your mind and say, "Oh well, I can live any way. I don't have to have things go my way to be happy and I can be flexible."

Lynne Namka, Ed. D. in "You Owe Me! Children of Entitlement" wrote:

"Some children have a personality trait of selfishness and feeling owed. The demanding child often focuses on issues of "It's not fair." He feels on an unconscious level that what happened to him was not fair. And, in a sense, he is "owed" because he missed out on basic nurturing, love, limits and structure. When early dependency needs were not provided, the child feels a sense of loss and shame that manifests itself in being angry. This child may go through life angrily trying to get others to make up for what his parents did not provide.

The type of child may react continuously to perceived small injustices in daily life. In effect, he is saying to other people, "You owe me. Pay up!" He can't get what he wants from his parents so he tries to get it from other people. Symbolically, continual anger can be a covert statement to his parents, "It is not fair. Give me my basic needs. Pay attention to me or I will blow up." Yet the sad part is that no matter how much is given to him it is as if he has a hole inside that can never be filled[41]."

When I minister to someone who has a chronic disease, I find that more times than not that the person has a sense of entitlement. They think that life has not been fair to them and they are wallowing in self-pity. Self-pity is different than being selfish. Self-pity is when we are feeling sorry for ourselves. We just want to wallow in our hurts and trials and think, "Oh woe is me, my life is worse than anyone else's. I have such a bad life." We can think, "Everything happens to me, I am such a victim." When we are selfish we are just thinking of ourselves and we want what we want. We have pride. We have selfishness. It is the "everything I" and "it's all about me" syndrome. All of this comes with a sense of entitlement. When we have a sense of entitlement, we think that we are entitled to get what we want. We are entitled to having everything go our way.

When we are selfish, when we feel entitled and when we are entertaining spirits of self-pity, some place in your life you listened to Satan and his kingdom and you got the mistaken idea that you have to have everything that you want so that you can feel good. We can add to that a mistaken belief that everything you do or everything that everyone else does or says should feel good to you all of the time.

You got the mistaken idea that you needed to get everything you wanted and if you do not, you are entitled to feel angry and punish others or retaliate against them. Maybe you just stay angry and disappointed all of the time.

We have a mistaken belief in society in general. It seems that people feel that they are entitled to getting whatever it is that they want. Somewhere along the line in our lives we have learned to be selfish and entitled. How did we get this way?

One way is that we emulate what we see our parents or caregivers do. For example, if one of our parents was controlling and selfish, we can learn that to get our needs met we have to be controlling and dominant and selfish in a relationship. We see others behaving in certain ways in order to get what they want and we emulate what we have seen our parents do.

It is common to man to do what our fathers did. Let's look at what the Bible says:

1 Kings 15:3 *And he walked in all the sins of his father, which he had done before him: and his heart was not perfect with the LORD his God.*

We may not want to do what our parents did, but familiar spirits are in everyone's lives. It is just the way things are. Until we recognize our problems and we purpose in our hearts to work with God to change them, we can be walking in the ways of our ancestors before us.

Dr. Namka wrote:

"Children who have experienced early physical and sexual trauma including neglect and rejection may develop narcissistic defenses to deal with their early pain. Spoiled and overindulged children sometimes are at risk for the narcissistic behavior pattern of wanting to control others. Children who are required to live up to high parental expectation of being charming, talented, intelligent, beautiful so that the parent's self esteem can be enhanced, are also at risk. This is particularly true when the parent is disappointed and rejecting when the child does not live up to their expectations."

What we can say is that this is a familiar spirit that has attached itself to the family. The family members have seen others behave in these ways and they continue on in the patterns. Unless we come to God and we change our hearts and our ways, we are going to be influenced by the devil to continue in the strongholds and the patterns of behaviors that our family was doing. We can be programmed and not even know it.

The problem is that we are in denial. We have blinders over our eyes and ears and we don't even know why we are feeling what we feel or how we are behaving. There are a lot of behaviors that indicate that a person is involved in selfish thinking. Behaviors that we would not even think are indicative of pride or selfishness.

For example...Did you know that being shy is a form of pride or selfishness?

It is actually a fear of man. When we entertain fears of what people will think about us and if we are being overly concerned about the opinions of other people, this can indicate that we are in idolatry to ourselves.

When we are shy, we are thinking about what others will think of us and how we look to others, and will others like us and what will others say about us.

The Bible says we are not be worried about the opinions of men, not to fear what men think about us or even what they say about us if we're doing what we know is right according to God. In fact, if we are striving to live Godly lives, we can expect not to be liked.

God never said that we are never going to have trials or tribulations on this planet. He actually tells us just the opposite.

Matthew 5:45 *That ye may be the children of your Father which is in heaven: for he maketh his sun to rise on the evil and on the good, and sendeth rain on the just and on the unjust.*

John 16:33 *These things I have spoken unto you, that in me ye might have peace. In the world ye shall have tribulation: but be of good cheer; I have overcome the world.*

Sometimes people think that because they are Christians that God has promised that they would have everything be the way that they want it to be and they would have everything that they would want. But that is not the case. Jesus tells us that even though we may have problems or tribulations, he can help us to overcome our problems.

Our joy comes from the Lord not from getting our own way.

Nehemiah 8:10 *For the joy of the LORD is your strength.*

Philippians 4:13 *I can do all things through Christ which strengtheneth me.*

Getting our own way in a situation will last a short time, but the joy of the Lord will last forever.

Psalm 35:9 *And my soul shall be joyful in the LORD: it shall rejoice in his salvation.*

Our joy is in the Lord and in our salvation. If we are thinking that people should say and act the way that we think that they should, and if they don't we can't be joyful, we are misunderstanding God and His word.

We can think that if people are not saying what we want them to say and doing what we want them to do, then it is our job to try and make them change so that they can fulfill our expectations. We pray for them and we try and manipulate them and control them so that they will change so that we can be happy.

It is hard enough to change when we are very motivated and we want to work with God to change

when someone is not looking to change, it is only .
their change of heart and mind and a miracle of
God that can change them.

A miracle is possible, but it is not too productive
to base your life on that happening. We have to
accept people as they are right now, today.

If we are waiting for someone else to change so
that we can be happy, we might be waiting for a
long time, maybe eternity. We should not base our
lives and our peace and happiness on what other
people do and say.

There is one person that you can try and change
and that is yourself. You can change and then lots
of changes can happen, but to expect someone else
to change so that you can be happy is like nailing
Jello to the wall. You are most likely not going to be
able to do it.

When we are trying to change everyone to be like
we want them to be, we are trying to be their God
and we are practicing witchcraft. It is selfish and
self focused and a very narcissistic viewpoint.

We can and certainly should pray for people
and have hope and faith that God will answer our
prayers, but people have free will and God will not
force any of us to do anything.

When we are selfish and self focused, we can
also be very unhappy. We can be seeking to control
everyone and everything so that we can be in peace
and be happy. We are not here to satisfy our every
earthly and fleshly desire, but to honor God and
live for Him.

Remember our scripture, be angry and sin not? We can say be disappointed and sin not. We can be disappointed that people don't say and do the things that we want them to do, but we have to deal with our disappointments with God. We have to decide not to sin in our disappointment. We have to be flexible and drop our expectations of everyone.

The truth is that if we don't deal with our disappointments, we don't seem to be able to get over our disappointments. They tend to turn into grudges.

This selfishness and self focus comes from the principality of the Unloving spirit. In other words, people do not know how to love others properly or how to accept love from other people.

We can be so focused on ourselves and so selfish that what we think that we want and have to have can lead us to be stuck in self-pity.

Here are some expressions of self while living in our sinful flesh:

- Self-justification - justifying everything that you want or that you think is right.
- Self-indulgence - Excessive indulgence of one's own appetites and desires. Indulging one's own desires, passions, whims, etc., esp. without restraint. (Addictions.)
- Self-pleasing - pleasing ourselves in every situation.
- Self-reliance - relying on ourselves instead of God.
- Self-centeredness - the world is centered on you first and foremost. (Narcissism.)

- Self-righteousness - confident of one's own righteousness, especially when smugly moralistic and intolerant of the opinions and behavior of others. This can be a religious spirit gone wrong!
- Self-pity - Pity for oneself, especially exaggerated or self-indulgent pity, feeling sorry for ourselves.
- Self-protectiveness - protecting one's self interest and not even considering anyone else.
- Self-assertiveness – being aggressive, rebellious or belligerence.
- Pride - a high or inordinate opinion of one's own dignity, importance, merit, or superiority.
- Selfish prideful living brings contention and strife.

Proverbs 13:10 *Only by pride cometh contention.*

Only when we are prideful will there be contention or strife or fighting. The Bible tells us what can happen when we are entertaining selfishness (envy) and strife:

James 3:16 *For where envying and strife is, there is confusion and every evil work.*

When someone is focused on their own desires and what they want and what they think that they have to have to be able to be content or comfortable or in peace they are in idolatry to themselves. They are in idolatry to their own desires.

Since we rarely can have everything go our way, we can become very discontented. These people can also be easily irritated and the characteristic seems to be that they don't deal with the irritation. They become angry and they don't know how to deal with their anger. They are upset if things have not gone their way and they don't have the skills to self soothe themselves or to take their peace. They don't think about God in the situation. They are trying to take care of themselves.

They are also entertaining a spirit of fear if things don't go their way. They do not see how they will be okay or happy. They are projecting doom and gloom into their future.

These kinds of thoughts and behaviors come straight from Satan and his kingdom. Remember, the bottom line is that they are not happy or in peace unless things are going their way. They become disappointed because things did not go their way.

Their disappointment leads to anger and they just simmer in their anger. They don't know how to be honest about what they are thinking and/or feeling, and they might not even know why they are feeling the way that they do. The bottom line is that they don't work their issues out with God and their thoughts and feelings are just buried alive.

Feelings buried alive never die. They are just buried alive.

This equates to denial. These people are in denial. Remember the acronym for denial "don't even NO that I am lying." They don't know that they are not being honest with God and with themselves and with others, they just know that they are not happy and things did not go their way.

They don't face their issues or take their peace, and think that they can live in peace, but they continue to want to work on making other people do what they want them to do. They continue on in their same programming and patterns and they want to do the same things, but they want a different outcome for their actions.

Being selfish is a trait that is sometimes hard to identify. Here is a list of some of the personality traits that can come with being selfish[42]:

- The person blames his faults on to others.
- Nothing is ever his or her fault.
- They are Insensitive to the needs and feelings of others.
- They don't seem to listen to you when you talk to them because they only care about what they think.
- They can Fabricate their personality to impress others and to avoid rejection.
- They can use sex or gift giving or anything to seduce you into doing what they want you to do.
- Low stress tolerance.
- They can be easily provoked into anger.
- They can be easily irritated.
- They can think that people are to be manipulated for their own needs, and for accomplishing their desires.
- They can reject and abandon you when you don't do or say what they want you to do or say.
- They can have a need to control situations, conversations, and other people.
- Often perceived as caring and understanding and uses this to manipulate others.

- They don't share their real feelings, emotions or their true thoughts.
- They can be very slow to forgive others.
- They can seem to hang onto resentment and hold grudges.
- Their true thoughts do not match how they act towards others.
- They can be convinced they know more than others and is correct in all they do.
- They can lack ability to see how they come across to others.
- They can be defensive when confronted with their behavior.
- They can get emotional, tearful. This can be about their frustration rather than sorrow or true repentance with change of behaviors in mind.
- They can be impatient and can seem concerned with getting what they want NOW— immediately.
- They can seem to be envious of any other person who is loved or highly respected.
- They are always the victim.

Remember, the person does not have to have everything on this list, but this gives you an idea of what to look for in this profile.

When we are very focused on ourselves or when things don't go our way, we can become very irritated. We can have a personality or a pattern in our personality of being irritated.

I call this the PRINCESS AND THE PEA SYNDROME. This is just like in the fairy tale that is called THE PRINCESS AND THE PEA. This is where the story is about a princess that was put on a pile of mattresses, and yet she could not sleep if you put just one little pea on the bottom mattress. She knew that she was sleeping on a pea even though she had ten mattresses over the pea. She focused on the tiny pea and she could not sleep.

This person gets very irritated by something that someone else does and they can't seem to focus on anything else. There can be a million other things that they can do and think about, but they focus on the one issue that irritated them.

They can have obsessive thoughts that focus on what the other person said and did.

Just like the princess that could not get comfortable or take her peace on ten mattresses, we focus on the thing that irritated or hurt us and we can't seem to get it out of our minds.

Here are some more examples of how people lie and manipulate, focusing on themselves, the me me me syndrome. They act like Mr. Good Guy or Ms. Good Girl, but what they are really saying is "I wear a mask or false front." "I give the right answer." "I say what you want to hear." "I say what will keep peace." "I manipulate to get the result that I want. I fabricate my personality so that I can get what I want."

They can use the *poor me syndrome* that can sound something like this: "I am the victim of this unjust system." "Everyone is out to get me" or "why does everything just happen to me" or "why is this happening to me" or "I have more bad things to deal with than other people." They can become a Victim that can sound like this: "I am the one who got hurt." "I will convince others that I was more hurt than the victim." "I will convince everyone that I am the true victim. I am the one that matters."

They can get involved in a Power play that can sound like this: "It is my way or the highway." "I will dominate and control others." "If things don't go my way, I am angry and irritated and I will do whatever I have to do have things my way."

They can have a personality of Entitlement that can sound like this: "The world owes me." "God should make sure everything goes my way. I am entitled to getting everything that I want." It is the me, me me syndrome. It is "Everything I."

There can be a Selfishness that sounds like this: "I do not care for others." "I want what I want when I want it." The idea is that I am the center of my world and I should be the center of the world for everyone I come into contact with.

There can be Blaming everyone else for their problems and it can sound like this: "I blame others so I can avoid responsibility for my actions." "I will not take responsibility for my own actions because if others would just do and say what I tell them to, everything would be okay and I would be in peace."

Denial can sound like this: "I do not answer questions when I know the answer is unpleasant." I won't allow anyone to talk to me about anything that is unpleasant about me. Secretiveness: "I use secrecy to control others."

Everything listed tells us that the person is not telling the truth. They are manipulating everyone and everything around them so that they get what they want. They are really lying. They are not honest. They are in denial and they are not taking responsibility for their true feelings.

They have a self focus that is causing them to look at everything through their own eyes, not through the eyes of God or through the eyes of others. When we are focusing on our own needs and our own desires and we can't be compassionate or empathetic about someone else's needs or desires, we are actually opening the doors to Satan and his kingdom and diseases. God tells us to do quite the opposite. God tells us that we are to love others as we love ourselves and we should care about other people and their needs.

Romans 12:10 *Be kindly affectioned one to another with brotherly love; in honour preferring one another.*

Philippians 2:4 *Let each of you look out not only for his own interests, but also for the interests of others.*

Matthew 7:12 *Therefore, whatever you want men to do to you, do also to them, for this is the Law and the Prophets.*

Galatians 5:14 *For all the law is fulfilled in one word, even in this; Thou shalt love thy neighbour as thyself.*

We know that God wants us to love each other and care for each other. He does not want us to be selfish. He wants us to think about each other.

John 15:13 *Greater love has no one than this, that someone lay down his life for his friends.*

Love is God's nature and love is what ultimately heals us. If we have true agape love for others it is very healing. God tells us all about how to love each other and how to have relationships with each other.

1 Corinthians 13:5 *love: doth not behave itself unseemly, seeketh not her own, is not easily provoked, thinketh no evil;*

Love is not selfish. In order to have a nature like God, we have to be able to be flexible and not be selfish and self focused.

If we care about other people and think about others and not only about ourselves, it is very good for our immune systems. It shows love and compassion and empathy. It releases good chemicals into our bodies.

Here is a blog article that I read that tells us just how important this is:

"Scientists have finally decided to officially research love and its effect on the body. It is difficult to quantify the capacity of this ethereal center for compassion, tenderness, wisdom and passion. But, there is more and more evidence to suggest that love is indeed good for you.

Years ago, it was discovered that when nurses bonded with cancer patients, if they gave loving support, the survival rate of the patients doubled. This spawned other studies. One quite famous study conducted at Ohio State University on heart disease involved rabbits, all genetically bred to develop atherosclerosis (hardening of the arteries) and heart disease. To speed up the disease process, the rabbits were fed a high-fat diet. To the surprise of the researchers, at the end of the study they found that more than 15 percent of the rabbits had no coronary artery disease. Their arteries were clean.

The researchers were stumped until they discovered that the rabbits with the clean arteries had all been positioned in cages at waist level. The graduate student in charge of feeding the rabbits apparently enjoyed her job. She had taken the rabbits from waist-high cages out daily to pet and play with them before their feeding. In the beginning, no one could believe it. So the study was repeated several times, each time with the same results.

The feeling of love brings chemical changes that alter the condition of the body. The rhythm of the heart is steadied, senses are enhanced, a sense of well-being is enjoyed, and immune system function improves. People in love get sick less often. If you have love in your life, no matter if it is for a sibling, grandparent, child, friend or partner, it is a precious gift[43]."

The bottom line is that when we are selfish and we are self focused and we are entertaining self-pity and we think that we are entitled to having everything go our own way: we can actually be making ourselves sick.

My favorite scripture is this:

Proverbs 11:17 *The merciful man does good to his own soul, but one who is cruel troubles his own flesh.*

Mercy is love. When we are loving and kind and we have compassion and empathy and the fruits of the Spirit are part of our nature, we are more likely to be healthy. If we are cruel, or we are selfish and envious and jealous, we can be making our own body sick.

Envy and Jealousy

This leads us into our next topic which is envy and jealousy and covetousness and lust. All of this goes along with selfishness. The Bible that warns us how dangerous envy is to our health:

Proverbs 14:30 *A sound heart is the life of the flesh: but envy the rottenness of the bones.*

This is very clear. God is telling us that when we entertain envy, that is the rottenness of the bones. We have lots of bones in our body, and the Bible says that when we have envy it will cause our bones to be rotten.

When you listen to Satan, and you are in agreement with envy and jealousy, (remember that every thought that you have is associated with a chemical release in your body), your thoughts are creating a chemical environment in your body that is causing rottenness of your bones. What does that actually mean? Well, your bones are where your immune system is manufactured. It is where your blood is manufactured. Your body's immune system can be impaired where you agree with Satan and you are in agreement with envy and jealousy. That is a pretty dangerous truth!

As Harold H. Benjamin, PhD, notes, *"Laughter in and of itself cannot cure cancer nor prevent cancer, but laughter as part of the full range of positive emotions including hope, love, faith, strong will to live, determination and purpose, can be a significant and indispensable aspect of the total fight for recovery."*

Our immune system needs all the positive things that come from God in order to be strong. Because envy and jealousy are main issues that cause God's people to be experiencing curses instead of blessings, I want to shine the light of God's word on this issue.

First, let's briefly define envy and jealousy:

Envy is a sense of discontentment or jealousy with regard to another's success or possessions; an inordinate desire to have [something] possessed by another.

Another definition of Envy: "Anger or discontent at the good fortune or possession of another." The word envy literally means "to look at with evil intent." The Greek Translation: "a painful or resentful awareness of an advantage enjoyed by another joined with the desire to possess the same advantage." So the spirit of Envy doesn't just want to gain, he wants the other person to suffer loss.

Envy is very selfish. (Remember, a cancer cell is selfish!)

When a person is listening to Satan agrees with his thoughts that tell him to be envious, he is actually looking at someone else who has something that he wants. When he sees the person has what he wants, he now has two problems. The first problem is that he does not have what he wants, which causes him great distress. The person feels entitled to have what he wants. The second problem is that the other person has what he wants.

Not only does the person feel badly because he does not have what he wants, he feels worse now because the other person has what he wants. He thinks that he would feel so much better if the other person would not have what he wants. And, in his heart he wishes that the other person would lose what he covets so that he could feel better.

"Misery loves company" is an old saying that means that if someone is having a bad time, they will feel better if they can marinade in self-pity and misery with someone else who has big problems also.

It is actually what the Bible calls the evil eye. The evil eye is this exact thing. It means that you look at what someone else has with evil in your eye. The evil is that you wish that you had what the other person has and that the other person would not have what you want.

There are many scriptures in the Bible that talk about the evil eye. The Heart of Envy: is the evil eye. It is a sin that begins in the eyes and longs to possess what others have.

The evil eye can be part of a pattern of thinking that leads the person into being envious and jealous. This can actually feel as if it is a curse, when the person wishes that you do not have to have what they want so that they can feel better about not having what you do have.

An example can be a woman who never had children. If you have children, you can tangibly feel her jealousy when you talk about your children. Not only does the person feel badly because she does not have children, but she feels jealous and envious that you do. Let's look at envy in more detail.

James 3:16 *"For where envying and strife is, there is confusion and every evil work."*

Please notice the word "envy" in this verse. It is taken from the Greek word *zelos*, and it can mean a fierce desire to promote one's own ideas and convictions to the exclusion of everyone else.

This word *zelos* is where we get the word zealot. I found this definition of the word zealot, it describes a person who is so fixated, obsessed, and fanatical to his own cause that others perceive him as an extremist on the threshold of becoming militant. If a person is a zealot, there is no question that he has made up his mind.

In the case of James 3:16, this word presents a picture of a believer who is so obsessed, gripped, and preoccupied with his own view of things that he can't see or hear the view of anyone else. In fact, his militant perspective has made him lopsided in his thinking. He never takes a softer line but holds out until all the other parties admit defeat and agrees with his point of view.

Therefore, the word "envy" in James 3:16 could be translated this way: "For where there is a fierce desire to promote one's own ideas and convictions to the elimination of everyone else..."

If this kind of attitude continues, it will naturally lead to the next step in this horrible sequence of events. This is where strife comes into the picture! When you are trying to eliminate everything that does not agree with what you want, you can get into strife. Another translation of this scripture is this.

James 3:16 *For where envying and strife is, there is confusion and every evil work.*

We can see that if we have selfishness and a self focus and we feel entitled and we want to get our own way all of the time, this leads to strife. Finally, where there is strife, every evil spirit is there to try and tempt you to get into every evil work. It seems as if we are falling into Satan's trap when we are selfish and self focused.

Moving ahead, jealousy is an English word that is etymologically derived from the Greek word *zelos*. B. Webster's Dictionary has these definitions for this word: 1- "apprehensive of loss of exclusive devotion;" 2- "intolerance of rivalry or unfaithfulness;" 3- "hostile toward one believed to enjoy an advantage;" 4- "vigilant to guard a possession."

Here is another definition: "Jealousy is a fervent desire to have things transpire as one desires." So, we can extrapolate that this can mean that we can have a fervent desire that things should transpire as we ignorantly or selfishly desire. We can want things to be our way and we can think that everything that we want should happen just the way that we want it to happen. This leads us back to the selfishness and the self focus that we have been talking about.

Did you know that being selfish and self focused is also being jealous and envious? In the Bible envy and jealousy is linked with selfish ambition.

James 3:14 *But if ye have bitter envying and strife in your hearts, glory not, and lie not against the truth.*

Envy and jealousy is linked with strife and conflict as shown in the following scriptures:

Romans 13:13 *Let us walk honestly, as in the day; not in rioting and drunkenness, not in chambering and wantonness, not in strife and envying.*

1 Corinthians 3:3 *For ye are yet carnal: for whereas there is among you envying, and strife, and divisions, are ye not carnal, and walk as men?*

2 Corinthians 12:20 *For I fear, lest, when I come, I shall not find you such as I would, and that I shall be found unto you such as ye would not: lest there be debates, envyings, wraths, strifes, backbitings, whisperings, swellings, tumults:*

Envy is also associated with deeds of the flesh or works of the flesh in the following scripture:

Galatians 5:19-21 *Now the works of the flesh are manifest, which are these; Adultery, fornication, uncleanness, lasciviousness, Idolatry, witchcraft, hatred, variance, emulations, wrath, strife, seditions, heresies, Envyings, murders, drunkenness, revellings, and such like: of the which I tell you before, as I have also told you in time past, that they which do such things shall not inherit the kingdom of God.*

Envy is also associated with anger, wrath and rage in Proverbs 6:34; 27:4

Proverbs 6:34 *For jealousy is the rage of a man: therefore he will not spare in the day of vengeance.*

Proverbs 27:4 *Wrath is cruel, and anger is outrageous; but who is able to stand before envy?*

There are a lot of examples of selfish jealousy in the Bible. I am not going to go over these, but here are just a few that you can look up on your own.

1. The brothers of Joseph – Genesis 37:11,19; Acts 7:9
2. Korah - Psalms 106:16,18; Numbers 16:3
3. Jewish leaders - Acts 5:17; 17:5
4. Zealots - Luke 6:15; Acts 1:13

Below lists examples of being selfish, jealous and envious that we can experience[44]: (Excerpt from thegracetabernalce.org)

- Jealous of another's possessions, wealth, assets – (greed, coveting)
- Jealous of another's position, placement, job, advancement
- Jealous of another's authority, power, leadership
- Jealous of another's recognition, praise, prestige
- Jealous of another's abilities, talents, skills
- Jealous of another's accomplishments, achievements, success
- Jealous of another's intelligence, logic, knowledge
- Jealous of another's personality, social standing
- Jealous of another's relationships, communication, intimacy, marriage
- Jealous of another's loyalties, devotion, attachments
- Jealous of another's age, youth, maturity, experience
- Jealous of another's looks, appearance, beauty, health
- Jealous of another's clothes, style, sophistication
- Jealous of another's opportunities, privileges, advantages, good fortune

When we entertain spirits of jealousy and envy, we are actually selfish and we are focusing on ourselves and what we want. We are comparing ourselves to other people and we are coveting what they have.

When we compare ourselves to other people and we see what they have that we don't have and that we want, it can make us very unhappy. More than unhappy it can make us very angry. More than that, it gives Satan a right to our lives. It gives spirits of envy and jealousy a right to our lives.

When we look at what others have and what we want and don't have and would like to have, if we let those thoughts guide us and if we agree with those thoughts, we are allowing the spirits of envy and jealousy open doors into our lives.

If we wish that the other person did not have what we want so that we would not feel so badly, that is the open door for the evil eye.

The thing is that if we see self centered selfish behavior, we can say that we can also be looking at envy and jealousy and covetousness and lust. The Bible tells us that if we are looking at envy alone, we are potentially opening the door to every evil work. Every devil can potentially have access to our lives.

Remember that the problems that we see in the people who have this problem can have difficulty moving on and forgiving and being flexible and changing their minds. They have difficulty taking their peace if they don't get their own way.

We see envy and jealousy and selfishness throughout the Bible. I mentioned several instances of these before. To continue I do want to share about one story and that is about Sarah and Hagar.

Sarah could not get pregnant so she actually encouraged Abraham to have a baby with Hagar. Hagar had a son. Here is what Sarah said in:

Genesis 21:9-10 *And Sarah saw the son of Hagar the Egyptian, which she had born unto Abraham, mocking. Wherefore she said unto Abraham, Cast out this bondwoman and her son: for the son of this bondwoman shall not be heir with my son, even with Isaac.*

She was now acting in a selfish way with envy and jealousy in her heart. She was filled with selfishness and murder towards Hagar and Hagar's son, Ishmael.

These very issues are seen in the world today.

We can ask ourselves, when you see someone who has what you want, do you covet what they have?

Let's use healing or good health as an example. Do you see someone who is healed and do you hear the thought, "Why did God heal them and not me?" I actually have had people say, "I am jealous of your healing."

This may seem innocent enough, but it is envy and jealousy and it is murderous. Inherent in that thought is: I wish that I had YOUR healing. I would feel better if you were not healed. I want what you have. I want your healing.

I have seen this spiritual problem a lot in people who have a chronic disease. They are selfish and they want things to go their way. They feel entitled to have things go their own way. They are simmering inside when things don't go their way, and they are envious and jealous of others who have what they want.

If you have a relationship with this person, your relationship with them can be okay if you don't have something that they want. But if you have or get what they want, in their hearts they don't wish you well. They are angry that you got what they wanted and it hurts them to see that you have what they want.

It can be your healing, your money, your house, your good health, or your marriage. It can be anything.

This is a good place to talk about what the Bible calls the *evil eye* in more depth. The Bible talks a lot about the evil eye. You can look this up in your Bible and study what this is all about.

We are going to briefly define this because I know that this can be a problem when we have chronic diseases. It is something that I have seen in people who have cancer.

When someone has a problem with an "evil eye", you can just feel that they are jealous if you have something that they don't have. They are upset.

They are so unhappy with their own lives, that they can't stand it if you get something that they wanted.

Evil Eye

What is an evil eye?

Mark 7:21-23 *For from within, out of the heart of men, proceed evil thoughts, adulteries, fornications, murders, Thefts, covetousness,* *wickedness, deceit, lasciviousness, an evil eye, blasphemy, pride, foolishness: All these evil things come from within, and defile the man.*

Deuteronomy 28:54 says that those with an EVIL EYE will eat their loved ones. They are concerned only for themselves.

Deuteronomy 28:53-54 53 *And thou shalt eat the fruit of thine own body, the flesh of thy sons and of thy daughters, which the LORD thy God hath given thee, in the siege, and in the straitness, wherewith thine enemies shall distress thee: So that the man that is tender among you, and very delicate, his eye shall be evil toward his brother, and toward the wife of his bosom, and toward the remnant of his children which he shall leave:*

Proverbs 23:6-7 says that one with an EVIL EYE says, "Eat and drink...but his heart is not with thee." He has no love for others REALLY; he is concerned only about HIMSELF.

In Matthew 20:15, the one with the EVIL EYE is jealous, selfish, and concerned about himself.

Here is a definition that I found about the evil eye.

"So the EVIL EYE is the BIG "I" and "SELF" of one's heart and DUPLICITY. It is the hypocritical deception of seeming to love God and others but in reality caring only for SELF."

How do I see this manifest in people's behavior?

Let's look at an example: Have you ever had

something good happen to you and you tell someone about it and you can just see that they are not happy for you? They may not say it straight out, but you know that they are jealous and they feel badly that you got what they wanted. They wanted what you got for themselves and they get that bad feeling inside of themselves and they don't mask it very well.

An example of this can be, let's say that you bought a new car. The person is trying very hard to not let you see how they really feel, but you just know that they want a new car too. They are upset that they don't have one and now they have another problem, they are upset that you do have one.

This is the evil eye. They look at you with lust and covetousness in their eyes. They wish that you did not have the new car. They don't say this, but it is what is in their hearts.

They are selfish and they are not thinking of you, they are thinking about themselves. They would like to have your new car. They, and their wants and desires are always on their mind. They are unhappy with their own lives, they are jealous and they wanted what you havev. They have spirits of self-pity telling them that they should feel really sorry for themselves because they did not get what they wanted. They have a sense of entitlement that they should have whatever it is that they want. They have anger against you, because you got what they wanted.

Do you see how every evil work tries to come into your life when you are very self focused? When you are selfish, you just can't see beyond what you think is going to make you happy. All of these evil spirits are connected and they work together.

Sometimes people want to impress you with the things that they have. They get their self esteem from what they own and how others feel about them. They may think that if they have a big house, a more expensive car and designer clothes, big diamonds and lots of money, they think it will make them happy. If they think that you have something better than they have, they listen to those spirits of envy and jealousy.

They now think that they won't feel better unless they have what you have, or you don't have it either. Seeing you have what they want brings their loss in front of their eyes.

The person, who is in agreement with these spirits and ways of thinking, is very comfortable when things go badly for someone else. When someone else has something good happen to them, it can torment the person who hears of someone else's blessings. They feel bitter towards the person who has blessings when they do not feel blessed.

The spirit of jealousy pops up and it can sound like this, "I wanted that! How come they got it and I didn't? Where is God?" Here is some more of what this thing can sound like, "I want the other person to lose what I want so that I don't feel so badly that I don't have it. I really wanted what they got and I felt badly enough about not having it, and now that they have it, I feel really badly. God, How come they got it and I did not?"

The person now has two problems. One if that they don't have what they wanted. Two is that someone else has what they wanted.

This is not an easy thing to recognize and admit. The problem is that if you don't admit things, you can't quit them. If you see yourself in some of these things, don't let the devil condemn you! Let God convict you! Be happy and be convicted that you are seeing your issues. When you recognize your problems, God can help you to quit these things. This is not what is in your heart anyway, it is the devil influencing you. You have agreed with Satan and his kingdom.

What can you do if you see any of these spiritual problems in your own life?

If you see this evil eye tell it to go, come out of agreement with it. Repent to God for entertaining these spirits and patterns of behaviors. Make sure that you wash with the water of the word and find out how God would have you think and behave. Next, you can purpose in your heart to exchange your old thoughts and behaviors with the new ones from God and His word.

God's Character of Love

The Bible tells us that God's character is love. One of the characteristics of love is that it is not envious or jealous or selfish. Here are scriptures that tell us about love. Charity (in the King James Version) is another word for love.

1 Corinthians 13:4-7 *Charity suffereth long, and is kind; charity envieth not; charity vaunteth* *not itself, is not puffed up, [5]Doth not behave itself unseemly, seeketh not her own, is not easily provoked, thinketh no evil; [6]Rejoiceth not in iniquity, but rejoiceth in the truth; [7]Beareth all things, believeth all things, hopeth all things, endureth all things.*

This scripture is very direct about what love is and what it isn't. Sometimes people can tell you that they are actively loving you, but they are really just being selfish and doing what they think will make themselves happy. This can be very confusing for people who have not experienced love and don't know how to give love or what it looks like when someone is loving them.

When someone does not feel loved or cared for, they can become envious and jealous when they see other people receiving the love that they want.

Envy also includes feelings of resentment, but it is rooted in the person's unhappiness or discontent. It is also rooted in doubt and unbelief; they don't think that God will take care of them. They can think that the things of the world are going to make them feel better or feel happy.

Feelings of dissatisfaction or not being contented with what we have can cause a person to become envious of those who have what they believe they need to satisfy or fulfill them. They can begin to desire the possessions or qualities that they see in other people. It could be their appearance, popularity, job, home, reputation, lifestyle, health, experience, and etc. The envy and jealousy that they experience can cause them to become angry and bitter.

As you can see, jealousy and envy and selfishness are destructive. They can ruin relationships and aspirations and hopes and dreams and they can make you miserable. They can keep you from trusting others and feeling secure about yourself. They can prevent you from being happy for someone when they get ahead or succeed.

These spiritual problems can keep us sick and dying. They can open the door to let Satan and his kingdom have access to our lives.

In order to overcome these issues in our lives, we have to recognize our problems. We have to go to God and repent for entertaining these problems. We cast out the evil spirits that have been influencing us. We talk to God all about how we really have been thinking and feeling. We tell the truth! We wash with the water of the word and we renew our minds with the word. And we exchange our old ways of thinking and behaving with ways of thinking that come from God and His word.

Matthew 19:26 *But Jesus beheld them, and said unto them, With men this is impossible; but with God all things are possible.*

It does not matter what your thoughts are what your behaviors are, or what your disease is. With God all things are possible.

241

—— CHAPTER FIVE ——

Cancer - After the Diagnosis

In this section I am going to deal with the spiritual issues that can evolve after a person is given the diagnosis of cancer.

After someone has been given a medical diagnosis of cancer many things can happen to the person's belief system. Satan can come around and try and influence them with more issues that are not good for their health. Let me detail some of these.

Fear: The word cancer evokes fear, so when a diagnosis has been made, fear is definitely part of the after-cancer diagnosis profile. Some of these fears can be: The fear of death, fear of not being able to take care of themselves, fear of doctors, fear of medical procedures, fear of side effects of drugs, fear of medical personnel, fear of pain, fear of never getting better, a fear of medical maiming and torture from the procedures that doctors advocate.

Some of the spirits that can gain entrance are spirits of fear, dread, death, destruction, infirmity and pain.

Other fears that can develop after the diagnosis. For example, the person can be afraid of getting healed and having to enter the same life that they had before they got sick. They can be afraid that they will have to resume their former life and responsibilities that they did not like before.

For example, sometimes they just don't want to go back to work. Sometimes they like the attention that they have because of their illness. They have never had so much attention in their lives.

Also, now they have a real and serious diagnosis and everyone is feeling sorry for them. People and family and friends are willing to cater to them, where they were not willing to do so before. They can be in agreement with fear of losing the attention that they have now that they are sick.

When you are in agreement with a spirit of fear, you can find that you have what psychologists identify as "free floating anxiety." You don't know how to handle stress in a Godly way and the consequences of that can be that you may find that you live in a state of fear and high stress, anxiety and panic. This weakens your immune system and helps to create an environment in your body where cancer cells can thrive and grow.

Another fear that can develop is a fear of going back to the doctor. Since the person already has cancer, getting into agreement with this fear can further weaken the person's immune system.

Another issue that can develop is that an Unloving spirit can be given strength in the person's life. Our diseases stem from separation from God, from ourselves and from other people. When we don't know how to have relationships with ourselves, we can find that we have guilt, shame, self hatred and self blame. We have allowed the kingdom of the Unloving spirit into our lives. When this happens, we can feel isolated and alone and separated from other people. We can feel separated from life, itself. This gives our immune system the message to shut down. If we are only getting our self esteem from our disease, we have a reason to hold onto the disease process. It can feel like we have to have the disease to have any attention. We can think that if we lose the disease, we lose the attention from family, friends and doctors.

Another thing that we can see in the person who has been diagnosed with cancer is double-mindedness. These people say that they believe God, but they are in idolatry to doctors, medications and medical modalities.

Here is what the Bible says about being double minded:

James 1:8 *A double minded man is unstable in all his ways.*

The person is believing in the doctors and all of the medical modalities that the doctors say can help them to live. Once the disease has been diagnosed, a spirit of fear can drive the person to do all kinds of medical things that the doctors recommend.

I have no problem with doctors, and they have things that can help us while we are working on our spiritual issues with God. But, who should we think of first? GOD! Sometimes people forget God and they spend their time having their faith in doctors and not in God.

Jeremiah 33:3 *Call unto me, and I will answer thee, and show thee great and mighty things, which thou knowest not.*

The first person we should think of is our God. We should call Him first, and last, no matter what else we are doing.

Medications: When you go to the doctor and they diagnose cancer, the medical community immediately wants to give you drugs, radiation and surgery. This can bring in a spirit of pharmakia and sorcery to your life. The fear is that if you don't take the drugs you cannot get well. The truth can actually be that if you take the drugs, you are sicker than you were before you took them. The drugs or radiation that is prescribed are sometimes so severe that they cause cancer themselves. The drugs cause fear if you take them, and fear if you do not take them.

The side effects from the drugs can be worse than the actual disease process. We have to learn to make decisions out of wisdom and knowledge and not out of fear.

Again, doctors and drugs can help us. But, always remember God and what He can do for you. Get an education! Research all of the modalities that the doctors are offering you. Make informed decisions about the treatments that you will choose to do.

Above all, work with God to uncover your spiritual issues and the roots to your disease. Work with God so that He can change you and transform you into the image of Jesus. In this way your body will have a healthy environment where disease cannot prosper.

Occultism: Idolatry becomes another spiritual element. The person who has cancer tends to have idolatry towards the doctors and the medicines that are supposed to save them. They may believe in God and be hoping for a miracle, but they believe in the doctors first and foremost. They tend to go to the doctor a lot and they depend on and get peace from the treatments that the doctors give them. Their hope is in the doctors; they hope that the Lord will bless their treatments and that they will be healed.

Their hope should be in the Lord and they should be seeking God just as diligently on what the roots to their disease are and walking them out as diligently as they are seeking medical treatment.

Another problem that we can see is that the person can be entertaining a spirit of death. A spirit of death and destruction can begin to be evident sometimes to the point of seeing that the person is not joining in on life. They do not feel safe, they don't do "living" things like having fun, or looking to the future or having hopes and dreams.

Proverbs 29:18 *Where there is no vision, the people perish.*

They have a vision, but it is death. We have to have a vision that includes life! We have to want to live and fight to live.

Another issue we can see is that an attention getting spirit may be invoked due to all of the attention that is being showered on the person. Sometimes family and friends are now focusing on the person as are the doctors etc. This can be the first time that the person has people focusing on them and giving them attention.

They can like being taken care of. This is a BAD habit to begin. Sometimes it is the only time that they have felt taken care of. The person can mistake the concern and attention that they receive from doctors, nurses, family etc., for the love that they desire.

The patient or victim, (they can feel as if they are victims) can think that people have hurt them. They can think that they are fine and they have done nothing to take responsibility for. They can be blaming their problems on other people and they think that they have had others who have abused them. They can feel that they are the ones that bad things always happen to and they can feel that they cannot have a good life because they cannot forget what others have done to them, what God has not done for them and what they wanted and did not get. They can feel that they cannot overcome what has happened to them in their lives and they don't want to live unless things go the way that they wanted them to. They are victims of the world, victims of other people, and victims of God. Everything is someone else's fault. It is the blame game, it is you God or the other people in their lives that has made me feel this way.

If you tell the person that this might be happening, usually it is news to them. They can think that cancer is just another thing that has happened to them. But the problem with thinking that way is that we can think that we are just victims of cancer and that God can't help us with this problem.

The devil loves to make people feel powerless and hopeless and helpless. If you believe the devil and you think that God cannot heal cancer, then you are the devil's victim.

When we turn our thinking around to God's way of thinking the cancer cells that have been thriving and growing in your body due to the toxic environment in your body will not be able to live. Remember, the thoughts that we have in our minds, are associated with a chemical release into your body. If these thoughts don't line up with God and His word, we are releasing chemicals that create the environment that these cancer cells love and thrive in.

If you have an intimate relationship with God and you allow God to change you and transform you, the environment in your body will change and the cancer cells will die.

Remember, you are not a victim. Take control of your thoughts with God and you and God can change your life.

Another issue we can look at is THE MOUTH. Talking about the disease can take over the person's life and focus and discussions. Talking about themselves and their disease is all that the person seems to think about. They talk about the doctor's, the next treatments, the pain, the disease itself, why their disease is so deadly etc. It almost seems that once a diagnosis is made the disease is the person's only interest and life. It takes over. Cancer takes over, essentially the devil takes over.

Hopelessness and Despair can also take over. The person has heard all of the verbal testimonies of death from their disease and they seem to believe it more than anything else. Doctor's reports can kill their hope. This is a different hopelessness and despair that happens before the cancer. Before the cancer their hopelessness and despair comes from being disappointed and angry that things did not go the way that they wanted them to go. They are hopeless because they don't see how they will make things go their way. They don't have flexibility to be able to say, even though things did not go my way, I can drop my expectations of life and others and myself and I can live for God and have a good life. Hopelessness comes after the diagnosis because the person does not see a way out of the disease of cancer.

Another issue to look at is the person's daily activities. Look at the person's daily activities, they sometimes look like they are already dead. It can seem as if the person is entertaining a spirit of death. The person is not really joining life. They are in agreement with their disease and it has become their whole life. It is their entire reality.

We have to live every day, hoping in the Lord. Hope in our hearts gives us a tremendous lift to our immune systems.

Another important issue to look at is SELF-PITY. They can say WHY ME? They can also get into testifying that their disease is the worst, no one has such a bad case, etc. They have had the worst life, the worst things have happened to them, and they are righteous in their self-pity.

They have self-pity but at the same time they are bathing in all of the attention that the disease has brought into their life.

A spirit of pride is also involved in this way of thinking. They are so self-focused and they believe that they are entitled to a good life and they believe that they are entitled to have gotten what they wanted.

Here are several other weapons Satan uses for those with a cancer personality:

Self-Centered Thinking: There can be a generational lack of nurturing, generational rejections and a fear of rejection and abandonment. They are in idolatry to themselves and if things do not go their way, they become angry and they simmer beneath the surface. They want things to go their way and they are not flexible.

Perfectionism: Trying to be perfect to get love and self esteem.

Performance: They can be performing to get love.

Fear of Man: Trying to please others to get and receive love and self esteem. Fearing rejection and fearing abandonment.

Lying: They tend to not tell the truth about their feelings. They don't tell the truth in relationships.

Below lists some things that the person needs to apply:

- Don't do things out of obligation with bitterness simmering beneath the surface, if you make a choice to do something, do it unto the Lord.

- Be honest with yourself and God by acknowledging and experiencing our feelings and then deciding to do the Godly thing!

- Get your identity from God and what He says about you, not from your performance and what others think about you.

- Do everything unto the Lord, not for performance or for identity or out of obligation.

- Pray about everything, tell God all about your feelings and then act on God's word.

- Learn about the kingdom of bitterness.

- Learn that not everything people do and say has to line up with your expectations.

- Learn to be flexible and to trust God.

- Learn to explore your feelings. Talk about your feelings. Pour them out to God and then deal with them. Honestly start to face your true thoughts and feelings. That is not to say that we act on these feelings or that these feelings are appropriate or accurate. We simply have to admit that they are there, recognize that they are there and not just accept them, but explore them and deal with them in a Godly way.

Cancer and Healing

So what about cancer and healing?

I know that God can heal any disease. I have seen people get healed from cancer, and so I know that God can heal you of cancer. No disease is too difficult for God to heal.

Matthew 19:26 *But Jesus beheld them, and said unto them, With men this is impossible; but with God all things are possible.*

Healing From God

We have described the character traits that can be seen in someone who has been diagnosed with cancer. The truth is that the person may not have all of the characteristics, but they have enough of them so that their immune system is so impaired that the cancer has a right to their life and their body.

When I minister to someone who has cancer. I know that each person is an individual. I can tell you that these are the character traits that these people can have in their personality and these are the traits that the medical community has seen and studied. I can also tell you that from experience, I have seen these issues manifest in these peoples' lives.

However, the most important point that I want to get across is that this information is just a starting point. God has created us all to be individuals. We are all unique. We all have different ancestors and different genes in our bodies and different familiar spirits and different experiences in our own lives. That is why I have to talk to each person and deal with their own unique issues.

I know that if I work with someone who has a disease like cancer, they may not have a clue about what their issues are.

For example, I have had people tell me that a minister told them that they have a problem with pride and self-pity. The person repented for these two issues in their life. They did not get healed. They did not know where these issues were in their personalities or their thoughts or beliefs or behaviors. I began to talk to them and teach them about where these issues hang out and hide. The next thing that we knew, God was showing them areas in their life that they did realize were coming out of these issues.

I have ministered to people who were losing hope because they had been a Christian for years and then they are diagnosed with cancer. They did not know why they had the disease. They had no clue what was giving the devil a right to their lives. They did not think that they had bitterness or envy, jealousy or fear. They did not realize that they were in denial or any of these issues that we have discussed.

When I spent time listening to them and talking with them and getting involved with the reality of their life, God revealed all kinds of things to them that were not lining up with Him and His word. They were lining up with Satan and they were in denial about what was really happening. They had no idea that they were jealous or envious or selfish.

God says that we are to be sanctified or changed or transformed into the image of His Son, Jesus.

I want to mention here, this is not just for cancer, it is for any disease.

The question we can ask ourselves is this, what changes should we make? And who should direct the changes? My answer is we want to think and behave like God.

In my opinion, God should be the director of our healing and our lives. What does God say about healing? Read His word, the Bible. The Bible tells us everything that we need to know.

Here is something that I would like to share with you:

The great Hasidic sage Rebbe Nachman[45] of Breslov (1722 - 1810) once made this generalization about disease and health:

"All the illness that afflicts people comes only because of a lack of joy. And joy is the great healer."(Pg. 39) Dr. Bernie Siegel offers a more contemporary perspective in referring to the "contentment factor." Siegel cites a long-term study dealing with the death rate among Harvard graduates, in which: "Those who were extremely satisfied with their lives had one-tenth the rate of serious illness and death suffered by their thoroughly dissatisfied peers even after the effects of alcohol, tobacco, obesity, and ancestral longevity were statistically eliminated."(Pg. 40) The two best-known mental and emotional factors that adversely affect health are stress and grief, especially if the latter is accompanied by loneliness. In the first half of this century, Walter Cannon discovered that heightened emotional states could stimulate the spleen, an organ that was later found to play a major role in the immune system.

What we have seen in this article, is that the way that we react to the events or the situations in our lives can determine how healthy our bodies are going to be. If we have stress, and we don't have faith in God, we are on our own. If we have grief in our hearts, and we don't have God, we are on our own. Without God, we are the only ones that can help ourselves out. BUT, if we have faith in God, we know that someone much more capable of handling our affairs can help us out. If we have faith in God and we know that God is going to help us and deliver us, our immune systems will work a lot better.

If we have faith and trust in God, instead of doubt and unbelief, our minds and consequently our bodies are going to have a lot more ability to be in peace and to have joy.

If we only have faith in man to help us or to heal us, we are trusting in a person. A person cannot even begin to know what our God in heaven, knows. Here are some scriptures that tell us the truth about God and man.

Romans 3:4 *God forbid: yea, let God be true, but every man a liar.*

Isaiah 55:9 *For as the heavens are higher than the earth, so are my ways higher than your ways, and my thoughts than your thoughts.*

Matthew 19:26 *But Jesus beheld them, and said unto them, With men this is impossible; but with God all things are possible.*

Here is an interesting and true story that shows us this kind of thinking in action.

How People Have Healed Themselves from Cancer & Other Illness via Their Mind[46]

My friend Jonathan Morningstar once cured himself of a terrible illness with a simple one line statement of gratitude. Jonathan got double pneumonia. Nothing seemed to help him. Then he felt inspired to write down one simple but potent sentence that he repeated every hour, recorded on audiotape and played back to himself, and wrote on signs which he hung around his home. He made this one liner part of his very being. And within twenty-four hours, Jonathan was healed. What was the one line he used?

"Thank you God for all the blessings I have and for all the blessings I am receiving."

Again, gratitude can shift everything. Just start feeling sincerely grateful for what you have. Look at your hands, or this book, or your pet, anything you feel love and gratitude for. Dwell on that feeling. Having a grateful heart to God is healing to our minds and bodies.

Psalm 100:4-5 *Enter into his gates with thanksgiving, and into his courts with praise: be thankful unto him, and bless his name. For the*

LORD is good; his mercy is everlasting; and his truth endureth to all generations.

John 11:41-42 *Then they took away the stone from the place where the dead was laid. And Jesus lifted up his eyes, and said, Father, I thank thee that thou hast heard me. And I knew that thou hearest me always: but because of the people which stand by I said it, that they may believe that thou hast sent me.*

Micah 7:19 *He will turn again, he will have compassion upon us; he will subdue our iniquities; and thou wilt cast all their sins into the depths of the sea.*

Psalm 103:2-5 *Bless the LORD, O my soul, and forget not all his benefits: Who forgiveth all thine iniquities; who healeth all thy diseases; Who redeemeth thy life from destruction; who crowneth thee with lovingkindness and tender mercies; Who satisfieth thy mouth with good things; so that thy youth is renewed like the eagle's.*

Does God Have an Ego Problem?

God tells us to praise Him and to be thankful to Him. There are many scriptures in the Bible that tell us this. Here are some of them.

1 Chronicles 16:8 *Give thanks unto the LORD, call upon his name, make known his deeds among the people.*

Psalm 30:12 *To the end that my glory may sing praise to thee, and not be silent. O LORD my God, I will give thanks unto thee for ever.*

Psalm 92:1 *IT IS A GOOD THING TO GIVE THANKS UNTO THE LORD, AND TO SING PRAISES UNTO THY NAME, O MOST HIGH:*

1 Thessalonians 5:18 *In every thing give thanks: for this is the will of God in Christ Jesus concerning you.*

Philippians 4:6 *Be careful for nothing; but in everything by prayer and supplication with thanksgiving let your requests be made known unto God.*

God does not have an ego problem! God does not want us to praise Him and thank Him because He has an ego problem. He knows that when we are grateful and thankful to Him, these thoughts will create an environment in our bodies that is conducive to health and healing. If we believe in God and we trust Him, we know that these scriptures are true for us.

Nehemiah 8:10 *The joy of the LORD is your strength.*

The joy of the LORD is our strength. Our strength comes from the Lord. We should not just be happy or joyful or peaceful when things are going our way. We have to have faith in God. It is important for us to know that no matter what is going on in our lives, God is real and we are on our way to eternity in heaven with God.

We can feel sad and we can feel all kinds of things, we can feel weak, we can feel sick, but we have to lean on God and remember this scripture.

Philippians 4:13 *I can do all things through Christ which strengtheneth me.*

God is the true source of our strength. We also know that scripture tells us this:

Hebrews 13:5 *Let your conversation be without covetousness; and be content with such things as ye have: for He hath said, I will never leave thee, nor forsake thee.*

God will never leave us, He loves us unconditionally and He is always there for us.

We also know that scripture tells us this:

Jeremiah 29:11 *For I know the thoughts that I think toward you, saith the LORD, thoughts of peace, and not of evil, to give you an expected end.*

God wants good things for us.

Here is one of my favorite scriptures:

Romans 8:28 *And we know that all things work together for good to them that love God, to them who are the called according to his purpose.*

No matter what is going on in your life, God can take the evil that Satan plans and use it for your good. And finally...

John 16:33 *These things I have spoken unto you, that in me ye might have peace. In the world ye shall have tribulation: but be of good cheer; I have overcome the world.*

1 John 4:4 *Ye are of God, little children, and have overcome them: because greater is he that is in you, than he that is in the world.*

1 John 5:4 *For whatsoever is born of God overcometh the world: and this is the victory that overcometh the world, even our faith.*

1 John 5:5 *Who is he that overcometh the world, but he that believeth that Jesus is the Son of God?*

God actually tells us that He will help us to overcome our problems and our tribulations.

When we know God and have an intimate relationship with Him, we can have the peace that passes all understanding.

Philippians 4:6-8 *Be careful for nothing; but in every thing by prayer and supplication with thanksgiving let your requests be made known unto God. And the peace of God, which passeth all understanding, shall keep your hearts and minds through Christ Jesus. Finally, brethren, whatsoever things are true, whatsoever things are honest, whatsoever things are just, whatsoever things are pure, whatsoever things are lovely, whatsoever things are of good report; if there be any virtue, and if there be any praise, think on these things.*

When we trust GOD and we have faith in God, and we have an intimate relationship with Him, He can lead us into peace. Remember, what is in your mind and spirit will be reflected in your body. If you truly know your God and rely on Him in times of tribulation, we will have peace in our minds and consequently in our bodies.

There is a way to deal with issues in our lives with God which leads us to peace instead of stress and anxiety.

Roger Dobson blogged "How to live to 114 (in theory)": Be religious—and have friends[47]:

Regular attendance at church or chapel can be as good for the health as jogging. A study at the University of Pittsburgh showed that weekly attendance at a religious service added two to three years compared with three to five for physical exercise and 2.5 to 3.5 years for people who take statins *(statins are a particular class of drugs used to lower cholesterol levels.)* "Regular religious attendance is comparable with commonly recommended therapies, and rough estimates suggest religious attendance may be more cost-effective than statins," say researchers. One theory is that it reduces stress levels or that the camaraderie increases the ability to cope with stress. A similar effect has been found for having friends.

Harvard University research shows that men and women who were less likely to attend church, travel, or take part in social activities were 20% more likely to die early than those who socialized the most. Those who engaged least often in activities such as work, shopping, or gardening, were 35% more likely to die prematurely.

I want to tell you about a scripture that can change your life.

Psalm 107:20 *He sent his word, and healed them, and delivered them from their destructions.*

This scripture tells us a lot about healing. It tells us that God sent His word – the Bible, and His word healed them from their destructions. It is the word that heals us. It is God and His word that can lead us into healing. It is a personal and intimate relationship with God that can lead us into healing.

Manage Stress: Think and Behave Like Jesus

The medical study that we just looked at said that we have to learn to "manage stress." The truth is that we have to learn to think and behave like Jesus did when He was on this planet. The truth is that we have to learn how to think and behave like our Father in heaven. Jesus told us that He only did what He saw His Father doing.

John 5:19 *Then answered Jesus and said unto them, Verily, verily, I say unto you, The Son can do nothing of himself, but what he seeth the Father do: for what things soever he doeth, these also doeth the Son likewise.*

Our goal is to think and behave like our Father in heaven and like Jesus did when He was on this planet. While we cannot see the Father, we can study the Son through His word. Since the Son ALWAYS does what the Father does, we therefore have a perfect model, Who is always available to all who love Him and are called according to His purpose.

We want to change the environment in our body so that it supports health and healing.

We do that with just what the scripture tells us to do.

Remember that Psalm 107:20 tells us that he sent His word and healed them and delivered them from their destructions. God sent His word so that we can be healed and delivered. The Bible does not say that God sent lots of medicines, special foods, operations, doctors, different alternative medical modalities or psychiatrists to heal us and deliver us from our destructions.

PLEASE NOTE: This is not to say that these things can't be used in our lives. But, God sent His WORD. It is the word that heals. When we hear the word and do the word, God can bless us.

I want to mention another scripture; because it tells us what else God wants us to do:

James 5:16 *Confess your faults one to another, and pray one for another, that ye may be healed.*

We are to confess our faults to each other. We are to talk to one another and to be transparent with one another. We should be honest with one another, and we are to pray for one another so that we can be healed. We are supposed to be in right relationship with one another.

Proverbs 17:22 *A merry heart doeth good like a medicine: but a broken spirit drieth the bones.*

When we are in peace and we have the joy of the Lord and the joy of our salvation, all of that is going to be like a medicine to us. God's word is a medicine to us. The second part of this scripture tells us that a broken spirit will dry up our bones, and our bones are the very place that our immune system is created. We communicate with God, Spirit to spirit, so if we have a broken spirit, we have a broken relationship with God and that can dry up our bones and harm our immune system.

Thinking and Vitamins

Isn't it interesting that one of the articles we looked at says this, "running a mile a day and taking vitamins won't counteract the effects of what goes on" inside of your thinking, "internally." What this says is that running a mile and taking vitamins won't counteract the damage of what you think and believe and do, if it does not line up with God and His word.

So if you have *stinkin thinkin'* or if your thinking is not lining up with God and His word, then all of the vitamins you spend money on and take and all of the exercise that you do, will NOT keep you from having a disease in your body or mind.

I found a study that I think will shed some light on this exact issue:

Schwartz GE, Weinberger DA, Singer JA, (1981 August) Cardiovascular differentiation of happiness sadness anger and fear following imagery and exercise. Psyhchosomatic Medicine 43(4):343-364.

The study is called Exercise and Stress (from EVOLVE YOUR BRAIN by Joe Dispenza, DC. (Page 274):

"A Yale University study conducted in 1981 involved actors and exercise. The researchers used actors because of their ability to access emotional states. The actors were divided into two groups. The first group was asked to make themselves angry. They worked themselves up by imagining frustrating and disturbing situations. The second group was asked to remain as calm, peaceful and stable as possible. Both groups were monitored for physiological functions, including heart rate, blood pressure, and respiration.

They were then asked to engage in various forms of light exercise, such as climbing a set of stairs. The so-called angry group maintained or showed less healthy levels in each health function. For the placid group, however, the benefits that we usually associate with exercise were truly evident. Only in this group, despite both of them doing the same exercise, did the exercise prove advantageous. Common wisdom held that exercise reduced stress, but our state of mind and state of being while exercising are just as important as the number of repetitions and sets we do to improve our health."
Isn't this what the Bible reveals?

1 Timothy 4:8 *For bodily exercise profiteth <u>little</u>: but godliness is profitable unto all things, having promise of the life that now is, and of that which is to come.*

God's word substantiates this very idea about exercise versus His word in this scripture. This scripture tells us where God and exercise fits into our lives. It tells us just what the study said that running a mile a day, can't help you too much if you are not thinking and behaving like God has told us about in the Bible. It is God and His word and His ways that promise us life here on this planet and into eternity.

I am not saying that we should not exercise, the scripture says that it profits little, and little is something and we need that profit, however little it is. But our eating and exercising can't help us if we are thinking and behaving in ways that don't line up with God and His word. It is our relationship with God that leads us into the kingdom of God and good health.

In summary, we know that food, exercise, vitamins and doctors can help us, it profits us little, but it does profit us. What really profits us or blesses us is an intimate relationship with God and Godly relationships with people and with ourselves.

So, we now know that even the medical community and their studies are lining up with what we know about God and His word. We know that there are definitely spiritual roots to disease. We know that our bodies will conform to what we think, believe and do. What we think, believe and do affects the health of our bodies.

The bottom line is this: The results of the study tell us that it did not matter how much exercise you did or how many vitamins you take, if you don't change the way that you think and behave, none of that will help you. The root to the disease, the way that you think and behave and if you don't change those things to line up with God and His word, the root to the disease would still be the same.

It amazes me how hard people work to learn about diseases and what to do when we are sick, when God tells us what to do in the Bible all along. I am not saying it is easy to work with God to be changed and transformed, but it is worth it. People are doing all kinds of studies to find out what God wanted to tell us hundreds and even thousands of years ago.

Godliness is profitable for us, all of the time and in all things. Not only does Godliness profit us on this planet, right now, but it profits us when we are in heaven too. Where do our profits or our blessings come from? Our profits or our blessings come from the kingdom of God. Here is another scripture that ties all of this together.

Romans 14:17 *For the kingdom of God is not meat and drink; but righteousness, and peace, and joy in the Holy Ghost.*

Godliness or the kingdom of God, is not meat and drink, or vitamins, or exercise or doctors or medicine, it is a relationship with God according to knowledge. It is righteousness and being a hearer and a doer of the word.

So, what heals us?

Psalm 107:20 *He sent his word, and healed them, and delivered them from their destructions.*

God sent His word and healed them and delivered them from their destructions. God does not say that He sent exercise and vitamins and doctors and medicine to heal us, He says He sent His word and that is what has the potential to really heal us. I am not against exercise and food and vitamins and doctors and medicine, exercise profits us a little and we need that profit, even if it is just a little. We need food to live. Sometimes vitamins can help us and sometimes we need doctors and medicine to help us while we are working on our issues with God, but if you want to be healed, really healed and delivered, we need God and His word. We have to renew our minds and wash with the water of the word.

Romans 12:2 *And be not conformed to this world: but be ye transformed by the renewing of your mind.*

God tells us not to be conformed to this world. He tells us not to be stuck on what we have learned in this world but that we should be transformed by the renewing of our minds with His word.

Ephesians 5:26 *That he might sanctify and cleanse it with the washing of water by the word.*

We want to be sanctified and cleansed by washing our minds with His word. When we renew our minds and we wash all of the un-renewed parts of our minds or our souls with the word, we will prosper and be in health.

3 John 1:2 *Beloved, I wish above all things that thou mayest prosper and be in health, even as thy soul prospereth.*

As you renew your mind or your soul by washing with the water of the word, your soul will prosper and so will your health. Your body prospers and you will have good health as your soul or your mind prospers and that is when we renew our minds with God's word.

The truth of the word is what sets us FREE. So, again the word is telling us that if you renew your mind or your soul and your soul will begin to prosper so will your health. Remember, what is in your mind or your soul, will be reflected in the health of your body. Interesting? Yes, but more than that it is life changing and life saving information to know. What does God want us to know about how to be a doer of His word? How do we do His word?

Galatians 5:14 *For all the law is fulfilled in one word, even in this; Thou shalt love thy neighbour as thyself.*

God wants us to have a relationship with Him and with other people and with ourselves— according to knowledge and according to His nature and His word. God is all about relationships. He wants us to have healthy, Godly relationships with each other and with Him. Disease has a right to our lives when we have a breakdown on one or all three of the following levels of relationship—our relationship with God, with ourselves and with other people.

REMEMBER: Our health depends on our relationship with God, with ourselves and with other people.

— CHAPTER SIX —

God's Prognosis vs. Doctor's Prognosis

I hope that I am convincing you that God's word can heal you. God can heal you. Don't listen to doctors who give you a doom and gloom prognosis, listen to God, who tells you that He sent His word to heal you.

The protocols of most doctors don't take God and His ways into account in their medical practice, and they don't really know about spiritual roots to disease. The only thing that they tell you is what they learn in medical school. Medical school does not teach people about their Creator, or His creation or His ways.

A Healthy Environment

How do we begin to change the environment in our bodies so that it lines up with health and healing and not sickness and disease?

I want to mention that it is important to take care of our bodies with good, healthy food and clean water. It is good to exercise and rest. But the most important thing that we can do is to address our spiritual issues and our relationship with God.

What we have to do is wash with the water of the word and renew our minds with the word of God. We have to seek an intimate relationship with God so that we will begin to change the environment in our body to one that is conducive to health and healing.

Ephesians 5:26 *That he might sanctify and cleanse it with the washing of water by the word.*

Romans 12:2 *And be not conformed to this world: but be ye transformed by the renewing of your mind, that ye may prove what is that good, and acceptable, and perfect, will of God.*

What should we be thinking about?

Philippians 4:8 *Finally, brethren, whatsoever things are true, whatsoever things are honest, whatsoever things are just, whatsoever things are pure, whatsoever things are lovely, whatsoever things are of good report; if there be any virtue, and if there be any praise, think on these things.*

Proverbs 15:30 *The light of the eyes rejoiceth the heart: and a good report maketh the bones fat.*

Good reports or good thoughts make our bones fat. Our bones are the very place where our immune system is created. So, when we think on the good things and things that are from the word of God, we are making our bones fat. We are thinking health into our bones.

Spirit, Soul and Body

We know that in our creation by our Creator God, we have been created to have a soul, a spirit and a body.

1 Thessalonians 5:23 *And the very God of peace sanctify you wholly; and I pray God your whole spirit and soul and body be preserved blameless unto the coming of our Lord Jesus Christ.*

Our soul consists of our mind, our will, our intelligence, our memories, our emotions. It is where we sift all of the information that we have coming into our lives to be able to make decisions and choices. Our spirit comes alive when we accept the Lord into our lives. God is Spirit and so when we communicate with God, we communicate Spirit to spirit. Our body is our mobile home that we use while we are on this planet to get around and to house our spirit, soul, and our body.

God created us to be very spiritual, physical, sexual, emotional and chemical in our creation. Every thought that we have is associated with a chemical release into our bodies.

When we have thoughts in our mind that lines up with God and His word and the Bible, we are in agreement with God which will create an environment in our body that is conducive to being healthy and free of disease. The opposite is also true. When we have thoughts in our minds that line up with Satan and his kingdom, we have a release of chemicals that produce an environment that can be conducive to sickness and disease.

The bottom line is that our bodies will be affected by what is in our mind and in our spirit. So, if we are sick and dying, the first place to look is in our minds and our spirits.

Your problems may be coming from right between your ears! The question to ask yourself is this, "What am I thinking? Whose thoughts am I agreeing with? God's or Satan's? Am I a doer of the word or a hearer only?"

Remember that God tells us to watch all of the thoughts that come into our minds. We are supposed to cast down the thoughts that do not agree with God and His word.

2 Corinthians 10:5 *Casting down imaginations, and every high thing that exalteth itself against the knowledge of God, and bringing into captivity every thought to the obedience of Christ.*

When you have imaginations or a thought that comes into your mind, that thought can come from one of three places. The first is that your thoughts can come from God and the Bible. The second is that your thoughts can come from Satan and his kingdom. The third place is that they can come from your own mind and your own beliefs, decisions, choices and evaluations.

The Bible tells us to have the word stored away in our hearts so that we can determine where each thought comes from. We can compare the thoughts in our minds with the truth that we know from the Bible. When we study the word, we are tucking the word away in our hearts so that the Holy Ghost can bring the word to our remembrance when we need to know it.

John 14:26 *But the Comforter, which is the Holy Ghost, whom the Father will send in my name, he shall teach you all things, and bring all things to your remembrance, whatsoever I have said unto you.*

Just because we have a thought in our minds, does not mean that we have to let it hang around. We don't have to agree with every thought that comes into our minds, we have a choice, we can cast them down. We can choose not to think any thought that does not come from God and His word.

Broken Spirit/Broken Heart

What can make us sick? What can hurt our immune systems that can create an environment in our bodies that can lead to sickness and disease?

Proverbs 17:22 *A merry heart doeth good like a medicine: but a broken spirit drieth the bones.*

A broken spirit, a broken connection or a broken relationship with God, will dry up your bones. Your bones are the very place that your immune system is made. If you meditate upon God's word and you think about good and pure thoughts that come from God and His word, this is your best medicine.

We can extrapolate from this that if we think about God's word and we are doers and hearers of the word, this will be like a medicine to us and it will give us the fat bones that we need to live healthy lives. Remember what God sent to us to deliver us from destruction? His word. Cancer is definitely a form of destruction and God's word can deliver us from any destruction.

The Truth About Satan

The truth is that Satan knows mankind very well. He knows how God has created His children. He knows what thoughts and behaviors that we have to agree with so that our thinking can create an environment in our bodies that is conducive to disease.

Our goal is to be in agreement with thoughts that line up with God and His word so that we have an environment in our bodies that lines up with health and healing. Our goal is to be hearers and doers of the word.

James 1:22 *But be ye doers of the word, and not hearers only, deceiving your own selves.*

My goal is to expose the devil and the thoughts and behavior patterns that Satan has influenced people to get into agreement with. These are lies we believe that can cause an environment in our bodies that is conducive to disease and even the specific disease of cancer.

If we find that we have a thought that is not in agreement with God, we can cast that thought down. We can refuse to be in agreement with Satan and what he wants us to think.

Remember, Satan knows all about us and God. He knows all about our creation. He knows just what thoughts to give us so that we will be in agreement with thoughts that can create an environment in our bodies that are conducive to disease.

We can't afford to let Satan lie to us. We can't afford to believe his lies. We can't afford to be in agreement with Satan and his kingdom.

Disease Prevention

If we, as children of God, receive God and His word into our hearts and we are hearers and doers of the word, we are going to be practicing disease prevention.

When we have thoughts in our minds that line up with God and His word and the Bible, and we are in agreement with God, we will create an environment in our body that is conducive to being healthy and free of disease. The opposite is also true, when we have thoughts in our minds that line up with Satan and his kingdom, we have a release of chemicals that produce an environment that can be conducive to sickness and disease. We can be allowing toxic and deadly thoughts and emotions to hang around in our minds. This can create an environment in our bodies that is going to let sickness and disease flourish.

Proverbs 23:7 *For as he thinketh in his heart, so is he.*

The Bible is telling us that the thoughts that we think, the thoughts that we agree with and we allow to hang out in our minds, will potentially determine the health of our bodies.

We are to meditate on the word of God so that it renews and washes our mind, setting ourselves up for living a healthy and abundant life. So, don't be afraid of cancer! As we talk about this subject and we learn about the thoughts and behaviors and patterns of thinking and behaving that can open us up to these diseases, just purpose in your hearts to be a hearer and a doer of God's word. Work on your issues and purpose in your hearts to come out of agreement with thoughts and behaviors that are conducive to an environment in your body that allows cancer to grow.

DENIAL: The Ostrich Syndrome

Do you have the ostrich syndrome? Do you bury your head in the sand like an ostrich would and just refuse to deal with the issues in your life? Are you in Denial? Are you the king or queen of de-nile? Are you following Scarlett O'Hara from the movie, *Gone With the Wind*? Do you think that if you don't think about something that it will just go away?

If you don't deal with the issues in your life in a Godly way, then the medical community has said that this is a personality trait that can open you up to disease. And one of the diseases that can have this as a root is cancer. I see people all of the time that push their issues underground. If something feels too difficult to face, they just push the issue away and basically refuse to deal with it. Sometimes I see someone who is so numb that they have no clue what their true feelings are. They just do not know what they are feeling. They just ignore their feelings and they go on, never really dealing with their issues with God.

This is a personality trait that leads to disease. I can say this without any question. It is one of the personality traits that can set a person's body up for disease.

According to leading alternative cancer treatment researcher Lothar Hirneise[48], *forgiveness is a primordial quality to develop for cancer patients.*

Also compare Dr. Bernie Siegel who writes: "I have collected 57 extremely well documented so-called cancer miracles. A cancer miracle is when a person didn't die when they absolutely, positively were supposed to. At a certain particular moment in time they decided that the anger and the depression were probably not the best way to go, since they had such a little bit of time left, and so they went from that to being loving, caring, no longer angry, no longer depressed, and able to talk to the people they loved. These 57 people had the same pattern. They gave up, totally, their anger, and they gave up, totally, their depression, by specifically a decision to do so. And at that point the tumors started to shrink.

This information gives us the insight that if we forgive as God tells us to, He can heal us. This tells us that when we have unresolved anger and resentment and bitterness, that this gives disease a right to hang out in our bodies.

The devil also knows this. His goal is to have people hurt us and offend us. He wants us to respond in ways that can make us sick and keep us sick. His goal is to have us marinating in the feelings that we have about the hurt and defilement that we feel. His goal is that we are never able to forgive and release the person who hurt us. Scripture tells us this emphatically:

Matthew 6:14-15 *¹⁴For if ye forgive men their trespasses, your heavenly Father will also forgive you: ¹⁵But if ye forgive not men their trespasses, neither will your Father forgive your trespasses..*

Ephesians 4:32 *And be ye kind one to another, tenderhearted, forgiving one another, even as God for Christ's sake hath forgiven you.*

When we forgive others, something happens to our hearts and our minds and consequently, something happens to the chemistry in our bodies.

It is not that God is saying, "I won't forgive you if you don't forgive others and I will be mad at you and hurt you because I am vindictive and I want to punish you." God loves us and has good plans for us. But, the truth is that He has created us in His image. God knows how He created us and He knows that if we do not forgive others, we will create an environment in our bodies that is going to let Satan have a right to our lives. When we don't forgive, this allows diseases to run rampant in our bodies and minds.

Sometimes people don't even know that they are angry. They don't know that they are holding grudges and resenting people and murdering them in their hearts. We can be so used to these thoughts and the emotions that come from the thoughts, that we are not paying attention to them. They can seem normal to us.

We have to remember that if we are not forgiving others it is just like shooting ourselves in the foot and waiting for the person that we are angry with to start limping.

Another analogy that I have heard is that when we harbor un-forgiveness, it is just as if we take poison and we are waiting for the poison to hurt the other person. It is not going to happen. It will only hurt the person who has the un-forgiveness and the bitterness. When we don't forgive, we are ultimately hurting ourselves.

I once read a testimony of a man who had cancer. He was told that he had days to live. So, he went home and he began to think, I don't care what happened on the earth in the past anymore, I truly forgive everyone. Then he began to praise God. He thought that he did not have to worry about money or bills or anything anymore. He thought that he no longer had to be stressed about anything. He knew in his heart that he was going to heaven and that he decided that he was going to start to praise God while he was here so that he would be used to praising God when he got to heaven.

The man's testimony was that God healed him and he lived without the cancer. He stopped worrying, and he forgave people because he thought that he was leaving the planet and he began to praise God. He had a drastic change in his thinking and that changed the environment in his body. God healed him.

Chronic Disease

There are several problems that I typically see in people who have chronic diseases. One of these problems is that they don't know how to feel their feelings. If they are angry, or embarrassed or they feel ashamed, or if they have any other feelings, they just don't know it or know how to deal with it.

They don't know how to identify their feelings, and they don't share their feelings.

God is all about communicating and sharing our thoughts and feelings with each other. Feelings are not wrong or right, they are just feelings. They tell us a lot about what we are thinking about. God tells us some information in His word that tells us how to handle what we are thinking and feeling. He tells us this in,

> **Philippians 4:6** *Be careful for nothing; but in everything by prayer and supplication with thanksgiving let your requests be made known unto God.*

God is telling us not to be anxious or worried about anything. Instead, God is telling us to pray. What is prayer? It is us talking to God and sharing our hearts and our desires and our feelings with God. Prayer is all about talking to God about anything and everything.

Dr. Henry Wright taught me to "Chew God's ear off." He taught me to keep talking to God about everything.

So God wants us to also talk to one another and share what we have in our hearts with one another,

> **James 5:16** *Confess your faults one to another, and pray one for another, that ye may be healed.*

Confession is good for the soul and also for our body, and anger can be unhealthy.

Ephesians 4:26 *Be ye angry, and sin not.*

From this scripture we know that God knows that we will have anger in our hearts or feelings. That is natural. However, if we do have these thoughts or feelings, we should not sin. We should share them with Him in prayer, and we can share them with others in discussions, but we should then choose to handle the thoughts or feelings in a Godly forgiving way that line up with God and His nature and His ways and His word.

Many of us were taught in our families of origin that showing our feelings or expressing our feelings was wrong. We saw our parents showing anger, but most of us did not see our families discussing feelings.

We grow up not knowing what we are feeling and we don't know how to discuss or share our feelings with ourselves or God or others.

(For more information pick up my booklet called: "Freedom to Feel")

Are You Past Feelings?

Let's look at some scriptures to see what I mean by asking this question.

Ephesians 4:17-25 *[17]This I say therefore, and testify in the Lord, that ye henceforth walk not as other Gentiles walk, in the vanity of their mind, [18]Having the understanding darkened, being alienated from the life of God through the ignorance that is in them, because of the blindness of their heart: [19]Who being past feeling have*

given themselves over unto lasciviousness, to
work all uncleanness with greediness. ²⁰But ye
have not so learned Christ; ²¹If so be that ye have
heard him, and have been taught by him, as the
truth is in Jesus: ²²That ye put off concerning
the former conversation the old man, which is
corrupt according to the deceitful lusts; ²³And be
renewed in the spirit of your mind; ²⁴And that ye
put on the new man, which after God is created
in righteousness and true holiness. ²⁵Wherefore
putting away lying, speak every man truth with
his neighbour: for we are members one of another.

This passage is so important. It helps us to
understand what our actual goal is. It helps us
to understand what the outcome of our personal
relationship with God can and should be about.

In this scripture, Paul is telling us not to walk
as the Gentiles walk. He is telling us not to live as
people who do not know Christ. Their lives are
marked by being past feeling. What does it mean to
be past feeling?

Let's look at what the concordance says: The
concordance defines this as being past feeling is
to cease to feel pain for. Here is a Short Definition:
I am past feeling, I cease to care and I become
callous. Another Definition we can look at is this:
I cease to feel [my] pain, I am past feeling, I cease
to care (suggesting sometimes despair, sometimes
recklessness). I can become callous and reckless.

The Christian is to be the opposite of being past
feeling. We are supposed to tell the truth about
how we really think and how we really feel. If we
are past feeling, we can be numb and unaware

of the truth that is in our hearts and minds. We are created in the image of God, and God is full of feeling, full of love, and full of compassion. Being past feeling is the characteristic of the old man, the old man dominated by greed, lust, and anger, fear and rejection. The Christian is to put on the new man, the new man who is conformed to the image of Jesus.

The way out of spiritual diseases is being conformed to the image of Jesus.

Conclusion to Healing the Cancer Personality

God tells us in His word that we are in a spiritual battle:

Ephesians 6:12 *For we wrestle not against flesh and blood, but against principalities, against powers, against the rulers of the darkness of this world, against spiritual wickedness in high places.*

God and His word is where we can go to learn how to fight our spiritual battles and win! However, we can learn much from the documentation and observations of the medical and psychological communities, presented in this book. They help portray the physical and mental manifestations of this spiritual battle. The experts in the medical and psychological communities have done an excellent job of documenting the physical and mental manifestations of our spiritual battles. Many of these studies and articles that have been documented here show us that what God has stated in His word all along, is true. The scientific community is just now starting to catch-up to Him.

We have learned that we are a triune being and the health of our body and mind reveals what is in our soul and spirit.

3 John 2 *Beloved I wish above all things that thou mayest prosper and be in health even as they soul prospereth.*

The thoughts, beliefs, and behaviors that you have will influence the health of your mind and body. Your body is speaking or showing what is in your soul or your mind and spirit.

Isaiah 55:8 *For my thoughts are not your thoughts, neither are your ways my ways, saith the Lord.*

What are God's ways? They are His ways of thinking, speaking, and acting; His beliefs, decisions, and actions; His motives, view points, and perspectives; His intentions, plans, and strategies.

When we are believing lies and we are thinking thoughts and choosing behaviors that don't line up with God and His word, we open up our lives to sickness and disease. When we are lining up our beliefs and thoughts and behaviors with God and His word our minds and bodies can work in healthy ways.

This is not the positive thinking that the world talks about, but it is Godly thinking.

This may seem like a lot of work, and it does take a lot of commitment, focus and determination. You are worth it! Your life is worth it! The wonderful thing is that with God; all things are possible.

Matthew 19:26 *But Jesus beheld them, and said unto them, With men this is impossible; but with God all things are possible.*

With God, there is hope for change. There is hope for us to exchange our old ways of doing things into the ways of God. There is hope to change our way of thinking and believing and behaving into God's way of thinking, believing and behaving.

This book has focused on the disease process of cancer, but these concepts can be applied to other diseases as well.

If we see ways of believing, thinking and behaving in our personal lives or in our ancestor's lives that don't line up with God, we can turn to God to help us to learn to love and accept ourselves; we can learn to face the truth and stop lying to ourselves; and we can learn to express our emotions and our needs, in a Godly way. We can learn to have healthy, Godly relationships; we can learn to resolve conflicts. We can learn to recognize our feelings.

We can change. The gospel is all about change in the healthiest possible ways—physically, relationally, and spiritually!

We can identify our beliefs, attitudes, thinking and behaviors that don't line up with God and His word, and we can begin to exchange these things with healthy beliefs, attitudes, thoughts and behaviors. Scripture tells us this:

Mark 9:23 *Jesus said unto him, If thou canst believe, all things are possible to him that believeth.*

The first step in changing is believing that things can change for the better in the Lord.

Closing Prayer

Papa God, thank You for Your Word, the Bible, that You have given Your children. Your Word is truth and Your Word is what makes us free. Thank You for Your mercy and grace and that I can come to You with confidence knowing that when I cry out to You, You hear me.

I recognize Daddy God, that my ways of thinking, speaking, and acting do not match Your ways of thinking, speaking and acting. My heart's desire is that I want them to be just like Yours. I want to think like You, speak Your words, and act, and behave and respond the way that You would. Daddy God, I no longer want to lean on my own understanding.

I repent that I didn't know how far away from You—I and my ancestors—had wandered. I recognize, repent, and renounce for doing things my way; and for acting and responding in ungodly ways. Help me to learn Your ways. I pray that You would help me to be transparent and honest and that I would no longer be in denial about the truth.

I ask You for forgiveness and that you would continue to open my eyes to attitudes, behaviors, and thoughts in my life that do not agree and line up with Your Word.

I decide today to stand on your Word, and lean not on my own understanding, but I choose to acknowledge You in my thinking, speaking and acting because I now know that when my thoughts agree with Your thoughts my body, mind, and spirit will prosper and be made whole. Because of the good news of Jesus Christ and by the power of the Holy Spirit, I get to be transformed and to be changed into Your image. Thank You for teaching me to walk and live Your way. Thank You that in You, and in You alone, there is true hope and life. I pray this in your Son's precious name, Jesus Christ of Nazareth. Amen

For more information or ministry, you can contact me at:

Barbara@freedomtofeel.com
www.freedomtofeel.com

Freedom to Feel
Pick up your copy today!

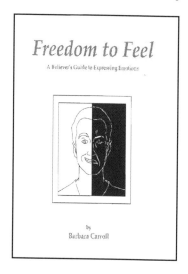

Your walk-out is important, so if you want to share your healing experiences with us, we would be happy to rejoice with you!

References

1. Book "A More Excellent Way" by Pastor Henry Wright. www.beinhealth.com
2. Freedom to Feel - Ministry Name and book by Barbara Carroll
3. Don Colbert, Md. He's Got the Cure, Charisma Magazine; November, 2003
4. Don Colbert, Md. The Dangers of Excessive Stress, Charisma; Jan/Feb, 2001
5. "Cancer Is A Message To You From Your Body http://www.alternative-cancer-care.com/AlternativeCancerTreatment.html
6. http://www.dailymail.co.uk/health/article-1028864/Your-personality-type-decide-makes-ill.html#ixzz0gGj5nsSA
7. http://www.dailymail.co.uk/health/article-1028864/Your-personality-type-decide-makes-ill.html#ixzz0gGj5nsSA
8. http://www.healingcancernaturally.com/hamer.html
9. http://www.alive.com/articles/view/19066/the_cancer_personality)
10. http://her2support.org/vbulletin/archive/index.php/t-18481.html)
11. http://www.healingcancernaturally.com/emotions-and-cancer-healing.html#positivethinkingserotonine
12. Full article at: http://www.healingcancernaturally.com/emotions-and-cancer-healing.html
13. http://www.healingcancernaturally.com/power-of-thought-to-heal-1.html (page 90)
14. http://www.healingcancernaturally.com/power-of-thought-to-heal-1.html

15. http://cancer.suite101.com/article.cfm/ personality_and_cancer
16. http://www.truestarhealth.com/members/ cm_archves10ML3P1A70.html
17. http://stevemehta.wordpress. com/2009/12/07/735/)
18. http://www.docstoc.com/docs/17632694/ Simran-Healing/
19. http://www.deborahkingcenter.com/ resources/advice/
20. http://www.leadershipcouncil.org/1/res/ brain.html)
21. http://www.socialproblemindex.ualberta.ca/ Socprobs.htm#Cancer
22. http://www.ivanhoe.com/channels/p_ channelstory.cfm?storyid=23357
23. http://www.alternative-cancer-care.com/ The_Cancer_Personality.html
24. http://www.journeyofhearts.org/transition/ pni_art.html
25. http://webspace.ship.edu/cgboer/ somatoform.html
26. http://www.tibetangoji.ca/health.html
27. http://www.alternative-cancer-care.com/ AlternativeCancerTreatment.html
28. http://www.healingcancernaturally.com/ resisting-alternativetreatment.html
29. http://www.healingcancernaturally.com/ real-life-healing-stories.html
30. http://www.healingcancernaturally.com/ real-life-healing-stories.html
31. http://www.alternative-cancer-care.com/ Lothar_Hirneise.html
32. http://ezinearticles.com/?Cancer- is-Not-a-Disease---Its-a-Survival- Mechanism&id=3906430

33. (89) http://www.healingcancernaturally.
com/power-of-thought-to-heal-1.html
34. http://www.healingcancernaturally.com/
real-life-healing-stories.html
35. http://www.livestrong.com/article/14669-
people-pleasing-personality/
36. http://www.alternative-cancer-care.com/
Cancer_Forgiveness.html
37. http://cancer.suite101.com/article.cfm/
personality_and_cancer#ixzzOolKSpoWj
38. http://www.quora.com/What-causes-
passive-aggressive-behavior
39. http://www.psychologytoday.com/blog/
passive-aggressive-diaries/200909/
backhanded-compliments-and-angry-smiles-
passive-aggression-de
40. http://health.groups.yahoo.com/group/
narcissisticabuse/message/3509
41. http://www.angriesout.com/teach9.htm
42. http://power2serve.net/Narcissism%20
Checklisg.htm
43. http://www.gotoloa.com/love-heals
44. http://thegracetabernacle.org/quotes/
Jealousy-Unrighteous.htm
45. (41) http://www.healingcancernaturally.
com/power-of-thought-to-heal-1.html
46. http://www.healingcancernaturally.com/
real-life-healing-stories.html
47. http://www.independent.ie/health/
case-studies/how-to-live-to-114-in-
theory-1504387.html)
48. http://www.healingcancernaturally.com/
emotions-and-cancer-healing.html

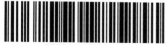

Made in the USA
Charleston, SC
25 August 2014